10-MINUTE CHAIR YOGA FOR SENIORS OVER 60

28-Day Program With Over 100 Illustrated
Poses For Flexibility, Balance & Mobility
Designed To Improve Posture & Lose Weight
for Beginners, Intermediate & Advanced

J.C. HARRISON
Gran Publications

Illustrations by ⊚ Jay.Illu

Disclaimer

This publication is provided "as is" without warranty of any kind, expressed or implied, including but not limited to warranties of performance, merchantability, fitness for a particular purpose, accuracy, omissions, completeness, currentness, or delays. The information in this book is for educational and entertainment purposes only. Efforts have been made to ensure that the content herein is accurate and up to date; however, the author and publisher make no guarantees concerning the accuracy or applicability of any content. Readers should independently verify any information within this book. The content of this book is not intended to be a substitute for professional advice. Should you require advice in a specific field, consult with a licensed professional who is qualified to provide such counsel. The author and publisher shall not be liable for any damages arising from the use, misuse, or interpretation of the information contained herein. The reader assumes full responsibility for their actions and the consequences thereof.

To My Mother

For allowing me to help you get back on your feet and proving to everyone that age is just a number and you can feel 20 years younger in less than 10 minutes a day!

– J. C. Harrison

Table of Contents

INTRODUCTION

Take care of your body, it's the only place you have to live.

— Jim Rohn

Y is for Yoga and Yoga is For You

Welcome to the only Chair Yoga Book you will ever need! You're not just picking up a book; you're stepping into a new arena of vibrant health and independence with "10-Minute Chair Yoga for Seniors Over 60". I'm here to guide you through a 28-day journey that's going to help you rediscover the ease of movement in your everyday activities, like playing with your grandkids or tackling a flight of stairs. Soothe the aches in your joints and ease the stresses in your mind, as well as embrace a newfound vibrancy that transforms routine tasks into joyful experiences, all designed to enhance the quality of your life as you gracefully navigate your senior years.

Let's talk about what's in store for you by the end of this book – real, tangible benefits that go beyond the pages of this book. Imagine waking up each day with an increased sense of flexibility. Those hard-to-reach shelves? Not a problem anymore. Your body is going to feel more fluid and younger, thanks to the strength and balance you'll gain from these chair yoga poses. We're talking about real physical health benefits here – the kind that makes daily tasks a breeze and keeps you moving like clockwork.

But let's not stop there. Chronic pain and discomfort – those unwelcome guests in your life – we're going to address them head-on. If you're skeptical about how gentle movements can bring about such changes, you'll be pleasantly surprised. Through these calculated movements, you'll learn how to alleviate this pain, giving you not just relief but a renewed sense of freedom. Imagine going about your day with less pain, feeling lighter and more at ease, that's what the power of chair yoga can do for you: manage and reduce discomfort.

Your mental wellness is crucial, as a healthy body needs a healthy mind. Stress and anxiety, those mental fog creators, are going to take a back seat. This program is your ticket to a calmer, more serene state of mind. We're talking about real mood uplifts, a noticeable drop in stress levels, and an overall sense of well-being that permeates your day. Picture yourself more relaxed, more in control of your emotions, and just... happier overall.

And here's the big one that seniors tend to love getting back: independence. This program is designed to boost your ability to do things on your own, with safety and ease at its core. We're aiming to keep you independent, spry, and capable of handling your daily tasks without a hitch. Imagine the satisfaction of managing your life on your terms, with a body and mind that are fully equipped to take on the world as you enjoy your golden years.

This program isn't just about sitting in a chair and doing a few stretches. It's about igniting a transformation that touches every aspect of your life. Alongside the physical practices, you'll find educational insights about each pose, helping you understand why and how they benefit you. This knowledge not only empowers you but also deepens the impact of each session.

As we embark on this journey together, it's important to recognize that every individual's experience with aging is unique. Whether you're a seasoned yoga practitioner or exploring chair yoga for the first time in your senior years, this program is designed with a spectrum of abilities and health backgrounds in mind. We celebrate the diversity of our readers, understanding that each of you brings a different level of mobility, flexibility, and experience. This book aims to meet you exactly where you are, offering modifications and variations to suit your personal needs and ensure a comfortable, rewarding chair yoga practice.

You're capable, you're ready, and you're about to embark on a journey that promises not just better health but a better quality of life. So, pull out your chair, take a deep breath, and get ready. Your journey to a more independent, healthy, and joyful life starts now.

Feeling a Little Nervous About Starting? We've Got You Covered.

Starting a new exercise program can be daunting, but we've got something special to help you **overcome fear and anxiety of starting a new exercise program.** As a thank you for getting this book, we're giving you exclusive access to an added bonus that will make your fitness journey smoother and more enjoyable.

When you sign up, you'll receive:

- A straightforward guide on how to ease your fears when starting something new.
- Tips to boost your confidence and keep your motivation high.
- How to discover exercises you love, that make working out fun and enjoyable.

Don't let fear stand in your way—sign up now and unlock this bonus designed to help you succeed!

https://geni.us/TheChairYogaProgram

How Chair Yoga Saved My Mom's Life

Before we dive into this book and get started, I want to share the short story about my mom and how chair yoga really saved her life...

Your journey with chair yoga will be unique in its challenges and its triumphs. Some of you are looking for just an overall healthy lifestyle (easy and fun to do), others aim to reduce or eliminate arthritis pain or post-surgery pain (like my mom).

When my mom came out of her surgery, she was worried she was not going to be the same person she was before, and she was right, she wasn't. Over time and with a bit of work, she became, stronger, more agile and I am not exaggerating here, but she seemed to be younger!

Chair Yoga saved her life. She is now keeping up with her grandkids (my little ones) and going for longer walks with her friends, she was even able to start swimming again. This is what chair yoga did for my mom, and it all started with less than 10 minutes a day.

This breakthrough wasn't just a personal victory for her; it inspired her friends to make the change too. As they witnessed her transformation, their excitement to make this positive change in their lives convinced me to write what would become this book for them, and now I am sharing it with the world for the first time.

<u>Here's a glimpse of what you can expect throughout this book:</u>

» **Getting Ready:** Dive into the essentials first. We'll explore everything you need to start practicing chair yoga in the comfort of your home safely and enjoyably.

» **The 28-Day Challenge:** The core of our journey, featuring over 100 poses fully illustrated spread across beginner, intermediate, and advanced levels. Tailor the program to your pace: follow a structured plan or pick poses that resonate with your comfort each day.

» **The Bonus Essentials:** We go beyond the chair in the final section, venturing into nutrition and meditation. It's a straightforward and easy-to-understand guide to nourishing your body and mind, complementing the physical practices.

Why This Book Matters

This program is about more than just physical exercises; it's a comprehensive approach to improving your overall quality of life as you age. From gaining flexibility to navigating stairs with confidence and ease and of course living pain-free, it's designed to support you at all levels.

Your Expectations, My Support

What can you expect? Progress, personalized support, and someone who understands your journey. If you need one-on-one help I'm just an email away, ready to assist you at no additional charge (jcharrisonbooks@gmail.com).

Thank You for Trusting Me

Choosing this program, and me as your guide, is a privilege I hold dear. Together, let's step into this transformative expedition.

Best wishes,

J. C. Harrison

C Harrison and I couldn't be happier to work with you on this

w journey you are about to go on. As you have already read, this journey

vith inspiration from helping my mother regain her fitness and health and

importantly helping her maintain it as she grew older.

What You've Purchased Is More Than Just a Book

You've just taken the first step with your purchase of the book, but I want you to know that you've gotten so much more! The Complete Chair Yoga Program is designed to be comprehensive and barrier-free, offering everything you need at no extra cost. Yes, you read that right—all the additional tools come free with your book purchase. I did this for my mother, and I'm doing it for you.

The Complete Chair Yoga Program Includes:

1. The Complete Chair Yoga Progress Tracker - $27 Value:

» Measuring your results is key in order to see progress, quickly and safely. I have a one-of-a-kind progress tracker that you will be able to use to track your progress throughout the length of the program.

2. Video Collaboration With Sarah Starr and Happy Yoga TV - $197 Value:

» Sarah Starr is a long-time yoga and chair yoga instructor who hosted her very own yoga TV show on networks like Amazon Prime. We have compiled a large collection of videos that are designed to go hand in hand with the poses and exercises you will have in this book. These videos will show you new ways and methods to practice chair yoga as you progress throughout the program.

3. The Chair Yoga Community For Seniors - $47 Value:

» Having a place where you can come ask questions and get encouragement or advice is what makes this the cornerstone of the program. We have built a fast-growing community of thousands of like-minded individuals who are looking to improve themselves and stay connected with others just like you.

4. Personalized Nutrition Plan and Meal Plan with Shopping List - $197:

» As part of the program, you will have a fully customized nutrition and meal plan created for you for the 28 days. Having proper nutrition can really help speed up your results and boost your energy, so I have included that for anyone who would like to have it.

5. One on One Personalized Support - $497:

» I am making myself available to you if you would like a slightly more personalized approach. Since I am unable to work with you in person one on one like I do with some clients, I will offer this via email for 3 months to help you hit your fitness goals. I am offering this cause I am serious about helping you reach your goals no matter what! Together anything is possible!

Total Value of $965

**TO GRAB THE REST
OF THE COMPLETE
CHAIR YOGA PROGRAM FOR FREE
SCAN HERE OR GO TO**

https://geni.us/TheChairYogaProgram

It's never too late to be what you might have been.

– George Eliot

CHAPTER 1
CHAIR YOGA MADE SIMPLE

Finally: A Chair Yoga Program That Gets You

Let's get one thing straight: yoga isn't just about bending and stretching. It's a powerhouse for your physical and mental health. Chair yoga takes it a notch higher for seniors, offering a cocktail of benefits tailor-made for your golden years. We're talking about increased muscle strength, skyrocketing flexibility, and balance that would make a tightrope walker jealous. But it's not just your body that gets a tune-up. Your mind gets a first-class ticket to relaxation town. Stress reduction, mental clarity, improved memory, and a mood lift are all part of the package. Imagine tackling your day with a calm mind and a body that feels like it's had a shot of youth juice. That's chair yoga for you.

Why Chair Yoga?

Think of chair yoga as yoga's more accommodating cousin. It's like yoga said, "Hey, let's make sure everyone can join in, chairs included!" Whether you're a spry 60 or a proud 90, chair yoga is your fitness pal. It adapts to your abilities, not the other way around. Got mobility issues? No problem. Chair yoga's got your back (and your knees, hips, and shoulders). It's all about making each pose work for you.

The goal? To get you moving, stretching, and strengthening – all while seated. It's so adaptable, that you'll wonder why you didn't start sooner.

Seated Poses vs Standing Poses

Seated poses in chair yoga are the cornerstone of this practice, offering a blend of stability, accessibility, and focused effort. When you're seated, you've got a solid base. This means you can concentrate on each movement, each stretch, without worrying about balance. It's about engaging fully in each pose, allowing you to gently strengthen and stretch your muscles, crucial for maintaining mobility and comfort in your senior years.

Seniors over 60 benefit greatly from seated poses as they are fantastic for enhancing your core strength – yes, even while sitting! They also work wonders for your flexibility, especially in the hips and lower back, areas that can be trouble spots as we age. But it's not just about the physical. These poses are excellent for improving concentration and mental focus as well.

Think of seated poses as your foundation in chair yoga. They're where you build strength and flexibility safely, setting the stage for more challenging movements. The beauty is, they can be as gentle or as intense as you need them to be. It's yoga that truly adapts to you.

Now, let's stand up and lean into the challenge with standing poses using the chair for support. These poses are your next step in the chair yoga journey, adding an extra dimension of balance and coordination to your practice. By holding onto the chair, you're able to try poses that might otherwise be out of reach, safely expanding your range of motion and capabilities.

For people over 60 years old, the standing poses taught in this book are exceptional for enhancing lower body strength – imagine gaining firmer, more stable legs and a stronger posture this in turn will give your balance a major boost. As we age, maintaining balance becomes crucial, and these poses are your secret weapon in keeping yourself agile and confident on your feet.

Incorporating both seated and standing poses, chair yoga offers a comprehensive approach to fitness and well-being. Whether you're focusing on deep stretches while seated or challenging your balance with standing poses, you're covering the full spectrum of movement, ensuring a well-rounded, effective practice. This is chair yoga at its best – adaptable, accessible, and incredibly rewarding.

The Real Deal on Chair Yoga: Separating Fact from Fiction for Seniors

Let's cut through the noise and bust some common yoga myths, especially those that might be holding seniors back from embracing chair yoga. This isn't just about setting the record straight; it's about opening your eyes to the truth of what chair yoga can offer you.

Yoga For Any Age and Any Body

First off, the myth that yoga is only for the young and flexible? Total nonsense. Chair yoga is positive proof that yoga is for every age and every body. It's designed to be accessible and adaptable, so forget the idea that you need to be a contortionist to get started. Chair yoga meets you right where you are, whether you find yourself as stiff as a pencil or as limber as a rubber band or you haven't touched or seen your toes in decades, this practice is designed to help you gradually increase your flexibility and mobility, no matter your starting point.

And if you're thinking "I'm too old to start yoga", I'm here to tell you, there's no such thing as too old. My mother started her chair yoga journey at the ripe old age of 77. Starting chair yoga now is like planting a tree today – the best time was twenty years ago, but the second-best time is now.

Get Ready To Sweat

Now, let's tackle the misconception that chair yoga isn't a 'real workout'. If you're thinking chair yoga is just sitting around and stretching a little, think again. This is a full-body workout that can strengthen your muscles, boost your flexibility, and get your heart pumping. It's a serious exercise, with serious benefits, all from the comfort of your chair.

Low Impact, High Results

Concerned about injury or discomfort? Let's put those fears to bed. Chair yoga is low-impact and gentle on your joints, but that doesn't mean it's a walk in the park. You'll work, but you'll work safely. And remember, you're in control. If something doesn't feel right, you have the power to modify it to suit your body.

So, let's throw those old myths out the window and embrace chair yoga for what it truly is – a powerful, adaptable, and enjoyable way to boost your health, no matter your age or fitness level. It's time to take charge, get moving, and feel great doing it.

Benefits Of Chair Yoga

✓ Flexibility and Mobility

In your golden years, dealing with conditions like arthritis, osteoporosis, limited range of motion, muscle atrophy, and balance issues is common. These can make everyday movements challenging. Chair yoga comes as a savior here, offering gentle yet effective exercises to combat these ailments. Through its targeted stretches and movements, chair yoga helps ease the stiffness and pain of arthritis, improves the range of motion, counters muscle weakness, and even aids in maintaining bone health. This results in smoother, more comfortable movements in daily life, enhancing your overall mobility and flexibility.

Strength and Stability

As we age, maintaining strength and stability becomes crucial, especially when facing age-related muscle loss and balance challenges. Chair yoga is a fantastic tool for tackling these issues head-on. The practice focuses on building core strength, which is vital for overall stability and balance, reducing the risk of falls—a common concern for many seniors. Additionally, chair yoga helps in combating sarcopenia, the natural decline of muscle mass due to aging, by engaging and strengthening various muscle groups. This not only aids in daily activities like lifting and walking but also contributes to a stronger, more stable posture. By regularly practicing chair yoga, you can enhance your physical stability and strength, leading to a more confident and independent life.

Posture and Balance

For seniors, maintaining good posture and balance is vital for overall health and independence. Age-related changes can lead to a stooped posture and balance difficulties, increasing the risk of falls. Chair yoga offers a practical solution to these challenges. The poses and stretches in this chair yoga book are designed to strengthen your core and back muscles, which are essential for good posture. By reinforcing these muscles, you'll likely notice yourself standing taller and sitting straighter. Furthermore, chair yoga enhances proprioception – your body's ability to sense its position in space, which is key to maintaining balance. Regular practice can lead to significant improvements in both posture and balance, reducing the risk of falls and contributing to a sense of confidence and autonomy in your daily life.

✓ Enhanced Breathing and Circulation

Chair yoga stands as a powerful tool for seniors, especially those battling respiratory conditions like COPD and asthma. It's not just an exercise; it's your path to deeper, stronger breathing. Each breath you take becomes more powerful, combating things like high blood pressure—a frequent issue as we age.

But there's more. The movements in chair yoga are your daily boost for circulation, directly supporting your heart health. They're your answer to easing symptoms of conditions like peripheral artery disease (PAD) and chronic venous insufficiency. This is real, practical health maintenance that works. Doing chair yoga regularly can lead to better overall circulatory and respiratory health, significantly enhancing your daily comfort and activity levels.

✓ Reduced Chronic Pain

For many seniors, chronic pain is a daily reality, often due to conditions like arthritis, osteoarthritis, and fibromyalgia. Chair yoga offers a gentle yet effective way to manage and reduce this pain. Its low-impact exercises and stretches work to relieve joint stiffness and muscle tension, common culprits of chronic discomfort. The mindful movements help to increase flexibility and mobility, leading to a significant decrease in everyday aches and pains. By incorporating regular chair yoga into your routine, you can experience a noticeable reduction in chronic pain, enhancing your overall quality of life and daily functionality.

✓ Reduced Stress

Stress, a common issue among seniors, can have far-reaching effects on overall health. Chair yoga offers an effective antidote. The practice's blend of gentle physical movements and deep breathing exercises is a proven stress-buster. Engaging in these calming activities helps lower cortisol levels, the body's stress hormone, leading to a more relaxed state of mind. This stress reduction not only improves your immediate sense of well-being but also has long-term health benefits, including better heart health and improved immune function.

✓ Improved Mental Focus and Clarity

Chair yoga is a valuable tool in combating age-related cognitive decline, a concern for many seniors. The focused movements and breathing exercises in chair yoga engage the brain, promoting neuroplasticity – the brain's ability to form new neural connections. This engagement is crucial in maintaining and enhancing cognitive functions like memory and attention, which can diminish with age. Regular chair yoga practice can also be a proactive measure against conditions like dementia and Alzheimer's, as it keeps the brain active and engaged. Additionally, the attention and concentration required for chair yoga are beneficial for improving overall attention span, helping to mitigate age-related memory loss, and maintaining mental sharpness. By incorporating chair yoga into your routine, you can support your cognitive health, ensuring your mind remains as flexible and resilient as your body.

✓ Boosted Mood and Overall Well-being

Chair yoga doesn't just benefit your body and mind; it uplifts your mood too. The physical activity involved in yoga triggers the release of endorphins, the body's natural mood elevators. Additionally, the meditative aspect of yoga promotes emotional balance, helping to alleviate symptoms of depression and anxiety. Regular practitioners often report a heightened sense of overall well-being, feeling more content, optimistic, and connected to their surroundings. This positive shift in mood can transform your everyday experience, making life more enjoyable and fulfilling.

✓ Improved Quality of Sleep

As the candles on the birthday cake increase, so often do sleep disturbances. It's a common issue for those over 60, with problems ranging from insomnia to disrupted sleep patterns. Here's where chair yoga steps in as a soothing balm. The practice's relaxation and stress-reduction techniques are a direct ticket to better sleep. By calming the mind and relaxing the body, chair yoga prepares you for a deeper, more restful night's sleep. This means waking up feeling more refreshed and energized, ready to tackle the day. No more tossing and turning, just peaceful slumber.

✓ Improved Quality of Life

Growing older can sometimes mean juggling multiple health issues, from chronic pain to reduced mobility, all of which can take a toll on your quality of life. Chair yoga is like a multi-tool, designed to tackle these age-related challenges head-on. By improving flexibility, strength, balance, and mental wellness, it touches upon various aspects of your health. The result? A significant enhancement in your day-to-day living. You'll find yourself more active, more independent, and enjoying life's pleasures more fully. Chair yoga isn't just about maintaining your current state; it's about elevating your everyday experience.

✓ Can Be Done Anywhere

One of the biggest perks of chair yoga, especially for seniors, is its sheer convenience. Mobility issues or lack of access to fitness facilities can often hinder regular exercise. Chair yoga breaks down these barriers. Whether you're in your living room, at the park, or even in a small apartment, chair yoga is doable. It's adaptable to your space and needs, ensuring that maintaining your physical and mental health is always within reach, no matter where you are. This accessibility is key to building a consistent, beneficial practice that fits seamlessly into your life.

Chair Yoga for Specific Conditions and Injuries

✓ **Finding Comfort from Arthritis**

If arthritis is your constant companion, chair yoga can be a game-changer. This gentle practice targets those stiff, painful joints, bringing much-needed relief. The movements in chair yoga are designed to increase circulation and flexibility, which means less pain and more mobility in those achy joints. Imagine bending your knees to play with your grandkids or curling your fingers without that familiar twinge of pain – that's what regular chair yoga can offer. It's not just exercise; it's a form of pain relief, tailor-made for arthritis sufferers.

✓ **Stronger Bones and Osteoporosis Care**

For those battling osteoporosis, chair yoga is a beacon of hope. This low-impact exercise is gentle on the bones yet effective in maintaining bone health. The weight-bearing poses in chair yoga can help in slowing down bone density loss, a key concern with osteoporosis. What's more, the improved balance and strength from regular practice can reduce your risk of falls and fractures. It's about keeping your bones strong and your body confident, one pose at a time. In support of this, a study examining chair yoga's benefits in older adults with osteoarthritis, a condition often co-occurring with osteoporosis, found it significantly improved physical function and reduced stiffness in men and women over 60.

✓ **Soothing Strategies for Chronic Lower Back Pain Relief**

Chronic lower back pain can put a damper on your daily life as you age, but it doesn't have to. By stretching and strengthening the muscles in your lower back, chair yoga can significantly alleviate back pain. These exercises increase spinal flexibility, which means less stiffness and more ease in your everyday movements. Think about getting out of bed or standing up from a chair without that wince of pain – chair yoga can help get you there.

Supporting this, a study done demonstrated its effectiveness for older adults over 65 with chronic back pain. The research found that engaging in chair yoga improved muscular strength and flexibility, which are crucial for managing chronic back pain.

✓ **Gaining Stability with Gentle Techniques for Better Balance**

Balance issues can be a daunting challenge, but chair yoga stands as a reliable ally, particularly with poses like Chair Warrior II. This practice zeroes in on fortifying your core muscles and sharpening your proprioception – your innate sense of spatial awareness. The result? A notable decrease in fall risk, a primary concern for many seniors. Chair yoga isn't just about enhancing physical balance; it's about instilling confidence in each step you take, giving you the steadiness and assurance needed for everyday activities

✓ **Lower Your Blood Pressure with Gentle Exercises for Hypertension Relief**

High blood pressure, or hypertension, is a silent adversary, a common and serious health concern among seniors. The chair yoga exercises outlined in this book offer a powerful ally against it, providing effective strategies to manage and improve your cardiovascular health. The stress-reducing and relaxing nature of chair yoga can have a positive effect on your blood pressure levels. By engaging in deep breathing and gentle movements, you encourage your body to relax, which can naturally help lower blood pressure. It's a peaceful, pressure-reducing practice that can be a key part of your heart health strategy.

✓ **Breathing Easier with COPD Using Soothing Techniques**

Coping with Chronic Obstructive Pulmonary Disease (COPD) often turns simple breathing into a daily challenge. However, the routines in this program are designed to alleviate this struggle. With a strong emphasis on deep, mindful breathing, they work to improve lung capacity and respiratory efficiency, ensuring each breath you take is more effective. Diaphragmatic Breathing or Belly Breathing is one of the exercise you will learn that greatly helps with this. This method transcends traditional physical exercise, focusing on achieving ease and comfort in every breath.

✓ **Ease Anxiety and Reduce Depression with Simple Exercises**

Anxiety and depression don't have to overshadow your golden years. Here's a bright solution: the meditative and physical blend of chair yoga. This practice is a powerhouse for releasing endorphins, your body's natural mood enhancers. A study found that chair yoga helped significantly reduce anxiety and depression when practiced regularly allowing you to shift towards a more balanced emotional state. Think of it as more than just a physical workout – it's a rejuvenating boost for your mental well-being, turning each session into a step towards a happier, more balanced you.

✓ **Restoring Flexibility and Strength After Joint Replacements**

Chair yoga proves to be a crucial companion in your recovery journey after joint replacement surgery. It offers a well-structured yet gentle regimen to help you regain strength and mobility while keeping pain to a minimum. Poses like Chair Pigeon Pose specifically target the recovery of hip joints, focusing on gently stretching and opening the area to improve flexibility and reduce stiffness post-surgery.

Tailored for your healing phase, this exercise (along with many others in this book) emphasizes movements that enhance, speed up, and improve your joint flexibility and improve muscle strength, all within a safe and comfortable range. By including poses like this in your routine, you'll likely experience a decrease in discomfort and an increase in overall functionality, contributing to a faster and smoother recovery.

✓ Chair Yoga for Balancing Blood Sugar and Managing Diabetes

Let's get straight to the point: for those of you over 60 tackling type 2 diabetes, Chair Yoga is not just an exercise, it's your key best friend. Think about it – just 10 minutes of seated yoga, simple, right? Here's the deal: research shows this no-fuss routine remarkably improves your glucose control and heart health. This is about making a small change with a big impact. It's practical, doable, and incredibly effective. Incorporate Chair Yoga into your daily routine and watch it work wonders. Remember, managing diabetes isn't just about medication; it's about taking proactive steps. Chair Yoga is one such step – easy to start, hard to overlook. It's your time to show diabetes who's boss. Strong, resilient, and determined – that's you with Chair Yoga on your side.

"

Every human being is the author of his own health or disease.

– Buddha

"

CHAPTER 2
SIMPLE CHAIR YOGA PREP
FOR SENIORS

Chair Yoga Made Simple

This chapter marks the beginning of a journey towards a harmonious blend of physical and mental well-being. Here, we focus on setting the stage for a transformative chair yoga experience, starting with preparing yourself mentally. It's not just about physical movement; it's about nurturing a holistic approach to health and well-being. We'll explore how to set realistic expectations, the significance of commitment, and the power of consistency in your practice.

Additionally, we will step into areas such as assessing your current physical condition, creating a safe and comfortable space for practice, and selecting the right equipment. This chapter is designed to equip you with all the necessary tools and knowledge to embark on this 28-day chair yoga journey confidently. Get ready to embrace a practice that not only enhances your physical health but also enriches your mental and emotional well-being, one day at a time.

Mindset

Before we pull out the chair and start bending and stretching, let's set the stage mentally. Mindset preparation is key, and it's where the true transformation begins. You're not just preparing to move your body; you're gearing up to shift your entire outlook on health and well-being.

First up, setting the right **expectations**. This isn't about instant miracles or overnight transformations. It's about gradual, consistent progress. Understand that every small step you take in chair yoga is a leap toward improved health and independence. The changes you'll see and feel may start subtle – a little less stiffness here, a bit more flexibility there. But together, they add up to something profound. Expect to grow stronger and more flexible, but give it time. Patience is your friend here.

Commitment is your next cornerstone. You've got a 28-day journey ahead of you, and it's essential to commit to this process. Think of it as a pact you're making with yourself. Each day, you'll dedicate a few minutes to your practice. It doesn't have to be lengthy; it just has to be consistent. This commitment is about showing up for yourself every day, and acknowledging that your health and well-being are worth that time. It's a powerful act of self-care and self-respect.

And that brings us to **consistency** – the real game-changer. Consistency in chair yoga isn't just about going through the motions; it's about building a habit and creating a routine that your body and mind start to crave. You'll find that the more regularly you practice, the more natural it becomes. It's like brushing your teeth – you just do it, and your day feels incomplete without it. Consistency in your practice strengthens not only your body but also your discipline and resolve. And the beauty of it? The more you do it, the more you'll want to do it. It's a positive cycle of well-being that feeds itself.

So, let's recap: Set realistic expectations – change is coming, but it's a marathon, not a sprint. Commit to the 28-day program – it's your commitment to better health and well-being. Be consistent – make chair yoga a non-negotiable part of your daily routine. With these mindset foundations in place, you're not just starting a fitness program; you're embarking on a journey of lifelong wellness.

With your mind primed and ready, you're all set to dive into the physical aspects of chair yoga. Let's get ready to embrace the change, one day at a time!

Understanding Your Present Physical Capabilities

Now, let's talk body. Before you dive into those poses, take a moment to assess where you're at physically. Be honest with yourself – are there aches that need nursing? Joints that need gentle coaxing? This isn't about discouraging you; it's about knowing your starting point. Understanding your current physical condition is crucial to tailor your chair yoga practice effectively. It's like setting the GPS before starting a journey; you need to know where you're starting from.

Creating a Comfortable and Safe Space

Before diving into the transformative world of chair yoga, let's focus on setting up the right environment. This section is dedicated to creating a comfortable and safe space for your practice – a fundamental step often overlooked.

Why is this important? Because your environment plays a crucial role in your chair yoga experience. It affects your concentration, comfort, and safety. This isn't just about finding a spot to place your chair; it's about creating a personal oasis where you can practice yoga without distractions or discomfort.

» **Quiet and Private Area:** Choose a spot where you won't be disturbed. This could be a corner of a room or a space where you feel relaxed and focused.

» **Enough Space:** Make sure there's enough room to move your arms and legs freely, stand up, and sit down without feeling cramped.

» **Good Lighting:** A well-lit area, preferably with natural light, is ideal. If natural light isn't available, make sure the area is brightly lit with artificial lighting.

» **Comfortable Temperature:** Ensure the room is at a comfortable temperature – not too hot or too cold.

» **Minimize Clutter:** Keep the area free from clutter to create a peaceful and safe environment.

Chair: Your Foundation for Practice

Selecting the right chair is like choosing the perfect dance partner – it needs to be just right for a harmonious experience. Your chair is the foundation of your chair yoga practice, so it's essential to choose wisely. Look for a chair that is sturdy and stable, preferably without wheels or too much cushioning, as you want to maintain a solid connection with the ground. The ideal chair doesn't have arms, allowing you the freedom to perform a wider range of movements.

The height of the chair is also crucial. When seated, your feet should rest comfortably flat on the floor, with your knees bent at a right angle. This position helps maintain proper alignment and balance as you move through various poses. A chair that's too high or too low can throw off your posture and even lead to strain or injury.

Clothing

Comfort is crucial when it comes to clothing. Wear something that allows for unrestricted movement – think stretchy, breathable fabrics. You don't need fancy yoga gear; just choose clothes that let you bend and stretch comfortably. Also, consider layers; a sweater or shawl can be handy for the relaxation portion of your practice.

Essential Props and Equipment: Utilizing Household Items

In chair yoga, you don't always need specialized equipment; many helpful props can be found right in your home. For instance, a sturdy book or a small, firm box can serve as an excellent substitute for a foam block, helping to bring the ground closer to your hands and offering support in various poses. If yoga straps aren't handy, a long belt or a scarf can work just as effectively for extending your reach and aiding in stretches. For additional comfort and support, regular household cushions or pillows can be used to prop up your hips or provide padding under your knees. A folded blanket is also versatile, perfect for extra seating support or as a cozy cover as you wrap up your session with some relaxation exercises. These everyday items are practical alternatives to traditional yoga props, making your chair yoga practice accessible, comfortable, and tailored to your needs without any extra expense.

Safety Tips

These guidelines emphasize the importance of a mindful and body-aware approach, ensuring that your chair yoga practice is both enjoyable and tailored to your individual needs and capabilities.

✓ **Breathe Fully and Slowly**

Embrace deep, conscious breathing in your chair yoga practice, which is especially beneficial for seniors over 60. Proper breathing is a cornerstone of yoga, offering physical, mental, and emotional benefits that are particularly pertinent as we age. As you move through each pose with ease, reducing the likelihood of strain, you'll find that mindful breathing not only promotes physical relaxation but also enhances mental clarity and emotional well-being. This approach is gentle yet effective, catering to the changing needs of your body. It helps maintain joint flexibility, improving circulation, and boosting overall vitality. Additionally, the calming effect of deep breathing can be a valuable tool for managing age-related stress and anxiety, fostering a sense of peace and contentment that enriches your daily life

✓ **Listen to Your Body**

Your body's signals are paramount. If a movement causes discomfort or pain, it's time to pull back. Yoga is about nurturing, not straining. Paying attention to your body's responses ensures a practice that is both safe and beneficial.

✓ **Keep Hydrated**

Hydration is crucial, especially for seniors. Drinking water before and after your yoga session helps keep your joints lubricated and your muscles functioning optimally. It also aids in overall circulation and body temperature regulation, which as we age becomes even more important.

✓ **Stretch Gently, Avoid Overdoing**

While stretching is key in yoga, overstretching can lead to injury. Approach each stretch with a sense of gentleness and caution, especially if you have existing injuries or conditions like arthritis. A mild stretch is more effective and safer than pushing too far.

✓ Twist Slowly and Carefully

Twists are excellent for spinal health but should be done with care. Never force a twist; your range of motion should be comfortable and pain-free. This approach helps maintain spinal integrity and prevents overstraining.

✓ Know and Respect Your Physical Limits

Being aware of your physical limitations is essential. If a pose feels too difficult, modify it or skip it. Chair yoga is adaptable, and there's always an alternative or modification to suit your comfort level.

✓ Limit Time in Each Pose

Long holds in poses can be more demanding and potentially risky, especially for beginners or those with certain health conditions. Start with shorter holds, gradually increasing as your strength and endurance improve.

✓ Focus on Regular, Gentle Practice

Consistency in practice is more beneficial than occasional, intense workouts. Regular, gentle chair yoga sessions are key to safely building strength and flexibility over time.

✓ Perform Mild Backbends Only

For those with back concerns, deep backbends might be overly intense. It's wise to opt for gentler backbends that offer a soothing stretch while being mindful not to exert excessive pressure on your spine. These milder bends help you to enjoy the benefits of flexibility and openness in your back, all while ensuring your comfort and safety. Remember, the key is to listen to your body and honor its limits, allowing for a nurturing and beneficial chair yoga practice.

✓ Avoid Pushing Yourself Too Hard

Pushing too hard in your practice can lead to fatigue and injury. Yoga is not about testing your limits but about gently expanding them. A mindful, moderate approach is always more effective and sustainable.

✓ Avoid Upside-Down Poses

Inversions (upside-down poses) are not suitable for seniors over 60, particularly for seniors who might have health concerns such as high blood pressure or glaucoma. Instead, chair yoga presents a wonderful alternative. It includes a variety of beneficial poses that can be performed safely and comfortably without the need for inversions.

My Mom's Pro Tips

As we embark on this chair yoga journey together, I want to share a few tips that really made the difference for my mom when she started Chair Yoga to help enhance your experience. These are simple but powerful ways to make the most out of your practice.

✓ Consistent Time

Finding a consistent time for your yoga practice is key. Choose a time that fits easily into your daily routine, whether it's morning or evening. Keeping a regular schedule helps in forming a habit and ensures that you're able to stick with it. It's about making yoga a regular part of your day-to-day life.

✓ Comfortable Environment

The place where you practice is important. Look for a quiet, well-lit spot in your home that's free from distractions. It doesn't have to be a large space – just somewhere you feel comfortable and can focus on your practice. Making this space inviting will help you look forward to your yoga time.

✓ Know and Understand Your Limits

It's not about pushing yourself to complete exhaustion, it's about extending your boundaries, gradually and safely. Adapting the exercises to what makes you feel safe and comfortable to help you get the best results.

✓ Free Online Coaching

To give you extra support, I'm offering free one-on-one coaching via email. If you have questions, need advice, or just want someone to check in with, I'm here for you. This coaching is a way to ensure you have all the guidance and encouragement you need to succeed in your chair yoga journey (jcharrisonbooks@gmail.com).

With these tips, I hope to help you create a fulfilling and regular chair yoga practice. It's all about finding a consistent time, setting up your space, and knowing that you have support along the way.

Before you continue!!
Make sure you download and fill out the The Complete Chair Yoga Program Progress Tracker. This tool will be essential for you going forward and in helping you hit your goals.

You can find it, along with the rest of the program for free, here:

https://geni.us/TheChairYogaProgram

As we grow older, our bodies need more loving attention and care, not less. Movement and gentle exercise can be a beautiful expression of that care.

– Unknown

CHAPTER 3
BREATHING AND
WARM-UP EXERCISES

Diving into Chapter Three, we tackle the essentials that set the stage for a successful chair yoga practice: Breathing and Warm-Up Exercises. We will guide you through a series of beginner-friendly exercises that are crafted for seniors over 60. These aren't just preliminary steps; they are the foundation for a safe, effective, and enjoyable yoga experience. Proper breathing techniques will enhance your focus and relaxation, vital for the entire session. Warm-up exercises are equally important, as they ensure your muscles and joints are properly warmed up and ready to go minimizing the risk of injury.

As we delve into chair yoga breathing exercises, known as **Pranayama**, remember this is more than just breathing; it's an art form that enhances both your physical and mental health. These techniques are specially tailored to improve lung capacity, reduce stress, and promote relaxation, essential for the holistic health of seniors.

DIAPHRAGMATIC BREATHING

Benefits:

This technique focuses on deep breathing, a powerful practice that not only helps to alleviate stress but also contributes to lowering the heart rate and stabilizing blood pressure. By encouraging a full exchange of oxygen, it nurtures overall respiratory health. Additionally, it plays a crucial role in strengthening the diaphragm, further enhancing the efficiency of your breathing.

Steps:

1. Sit comfortably in a chair with your feet flat on the floor.

2. Place one hand on your chest and the other on your abdomen.

3. Inhale deeply through your nose, allowing your abdomen to rise more than your chest.

4. Exhale slowly through your mouth, feeling your abdomen fall.

5. Repeat this process for 1-3 minutes, focusing on deep, even breaths.

Benefits:

Cultivates greater lung capacity and boosts respiratory efficiency. This technique serves as a calming and grounding force, effectively clearing the mind and diminishing stress. It's also instrumental in sharpening focus and enhancing mindfulness, contributing to overall mental clarity and well-being.

Steps:

1. Sit or lie down in a comfortable position.

2. Inhale deeply, first filling your abdomen, then your mid-chest, and finally the upper chest.

3. Exhale slowly and fully, reversing the order: empty the upper chest, mid-chest, and finally the abdomen.

4. Continue this pattern for several breath cycles, paying attention to each part of your breath.

Ocean Breath
(Ujjayi Pranayama)

Benefits:

This breath technique is a catalyst for generating internal warmth, essential for centering and sharpening mental focus. It plays a key role in harmonizing your breath with yoga movements, creating a seamless flow. Additionally, Ujjayi Pranayama is effective in soothing the nervous system and decelerating the breath rate, fostering a sense of deep relaxation and tranquility.

Steps:

1. Sit comfortably with your spine straight.

2. Inhale deeply through your nose.

3. Exhale through your nose while constricting the back of your throat, producing a soft ocean-like sound.

4. Continue this breathing, making your inhales and exhales long and steady.

Benefits:

This technique is celebrated for its ability to harmonize the left and right hemispheres of the brain. It plays a pivotal role in tranquilizing the mind, mitigating anxiety, and sharpening mental focus. Additionally, it offers significant benefits for respiratory health, enhancing overall breathing efficiency.

Steps:

1. Sit comfortably with a straight spine.

2. Place your left hand on your knee.

3. Use your right thumb to close your right nostril and inhale slowly through your left nostril.

4. Close your left nostril with your ring finger, release your right nostril, and exhale.

5. Inhale through the right nostril, close it, and exhale through the left.

6. Continue this alternating pattern for several minutes.

LION'S BREATH

Benefits:

Calmly soothes tension in the chest and face, and is celebrated for its revitalizing effects. It plays a significant role in easing stress and boosting circulation. Additionally, it is beneficial for throat health and enhances vocal flexibility, offering a holistic approach to well-being.

Steps:

1. Sit comfortably, inhaling deeply through your nose.

2. Exhale forcefully through your mouth, sticking out your tongue and making a 'ha' sound.

3. As you exhale, open your eyes wide and stretch the muscles of your face.

4. Repeat several times.

Benefits:

As implied by its name, this technique imparts a cooling sensation throughout the body and mind. It's particularly effective in diminishing stress and soothing feelings of anger and frustration. Additionally, it plays a crucial role in regulating body temperature, making it especially valuable during hot weather or following intense physical activity.

1   2   3

Steps:

1. Sit comfortably with your eyes closed.

2. Curl your tongue lengthwise and protrude it slightly past your lips.

3. Inhale through your curled tongue like sipping through a straw.

4. Close your mouth, exhaling through your nose.

5. Repeat for several breaths.

Box Breathing

Benefits:

This technique excels in stress management, as it aids in calming and stabilizing the autonomic nervous system. It also enhances concentration and sharpens focus. It's particularly valuable in high-stress scenarios or for individuals managing anxiety, providing a sense of balance and tranquility.

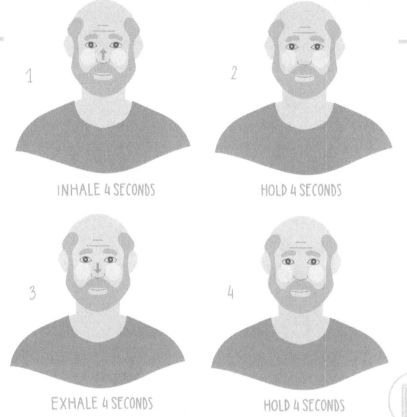

1

INHALE 4 SECONDS

2

HOLD 4 SECONDS

3

EXHALE 4 SECONDS

4

HOLD 4 SECONDS

Steps:

1. Sit upright in a relaxed position.

2. Inhale for a count of four.

3. Hold your breath for another count of four.

4. Exhale slowly for a count of four.

5. Hold your breath again for a count of four.

6. Repeat this 'box' pattern for several minutes.

Warm-up exercises and stretches help wake up the body, lubricate the joints, and ensure your chair yoga session is as safe as possible. By doing small movements you can help prepare your muscles and joints through activity similar to the poses you will be doing. This will help prevent injury and also allow you to get more from your actual chair yoga session.

Wrist & Ankle Rotation:

Rotate your wrists and ankles slowly in both directions. This helps to loosen the joints and improve circulation.

Gentle Torso Twists:

Sit upright with your feet flat on the floor. Place your hands on your knees. Gently twist your torso to the right, then to the left, warming up the spine.

Side Neck Stretch:

Drop your right ear towards your right shoulder gently, then switch to the left side. This stretch helps to release tension in the neck muscles.

Shoulder Stretch:

Bring your right arm across your body, using your left hand to press it gently towards your chest. Switch arms after a few breaths.

Toe and Heel Lifts:

With your feet flat on the floor, lift your toes while keeping your heels down, then lift your heels while keeping your toes down. This exercise warms up the feet and calves.

Gentle Backbend:

Place your hands on the back of your hips, gently arch your spine, and look slightly upwards, opening up the chest and front of the body.

Seated Neck Rolls:

Sit straight and gently lower your chin to your chest, then slowly roll your head in a circle, first to the right, then back and to the left. Repeat this motion three times, then switch directions.

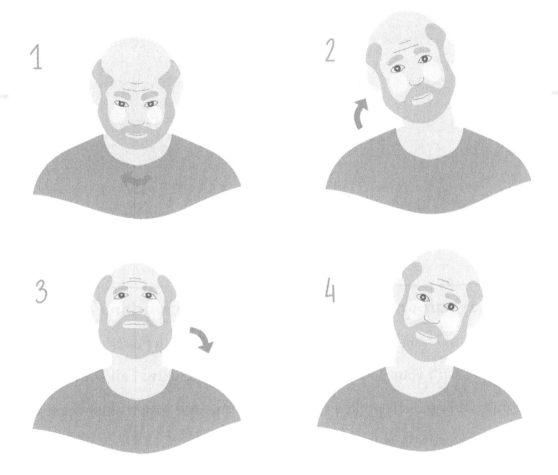

Be patient with yourself. Self-growth is tender; it's holy ground. There's no greater investment.

– Stephen Covey

———— **Stay Safe and Steady with Our Fall Prevention Guide!** ————

We know that maintaining balance and preventing falls is a top priority, especially as we age. That's why, along with your book, we're including **an exclusive Fall Prevention Guide** as a special bonus. This guide is packed with practical tips and easy-to-follow exercises to help you stay safe and steady on your feet.

Don't miss out on this essential bonus—sign up now and take control of your safety with our Fall Prevention Guide!

https://geni.us/TheChairYogaProgram

CHAPTER 4
BEGINNER 28-DAY CHAIR YOGA CHALLENGE

Welcome to Chapter Four, where we delve into beginner-friendly chair yoga poses specifically tailored for seniors. This chapter is all about empowering you with chair yoga poses that enhance flexibility, bolster strength, and improve balance – crucial for your golden years. You'll find each pose accompanied by clear, step-by-step instructions and illustrations as well as tips to ensure you're practicing safely and effectively. Whether you're aiming to ease joint pain, boost circulation, or maintain mental sharpness, these poses are designed with your needs in mind.

Our unique approach allows you to select from two different 28 day programs. Firstly we will review all the poses that are part of the beginner section and then at the end of this chapter you will be able to select which 28 day program you would like to begin: structured or flexible. Either challenge provides a great way to establish a consistent routine, allowing you to experience the health and wellness benefits of regular chair yoga practice. Whichever path you choose, you're on your way to a more mobile, balanced, and joyful life.

The 28-Day Beginner challenge can be found on page 90.

POSES FOR BETTER POSTURE

Targeted Areas:

Neck muscles.

Benefits:

This gentle exercise is designed for seniors to relieve neck tension and improve flexibility. By focusing on the neck muscles, it offers a soothing stretch that can enhance mobility and comfort in the neck area.

Safety Precautions:

- Perform movements gently to avoid strain.
- If you experience dizziness, pause and return to a neutral position.

Steps:

1. Begin by sitting in a comfortable chair with your spine aligned and upright. This posture ensures a safe foundation for the exercise.

2. Slowly tilt your head forward, guiding your chin towards your chest. This initial movement starts the stretch and begins to release tension in the neck.

3. Gently roll your head to the right, aiming to bring your ear closer to your shoulder. This action stretches the side neck muscles, aiding in flexibility.

4. Continue the motion by rolling your head backward and then to the left, completing a smooth, circular movement. This sequence helps to evenly distribute the stretch across the neck muscles.

5. Perform 3-5 rolls in each direction, moving at a pace that feels comfortable and safe. Ensure each roll is performed gently to avoid any strain.

SHOULDER SHRUGS

Targeted Areas:
Shoulders and upper back.

Benefits:

Excellent for relieving tension in the shoulders and neck, while improving upper body mobility. This simple yet powerful movement targets the shoulders and upper back, promoting relaxation and flexibility in these areas.

Safety Precautions:

- Move slowly and avoid overexerting the shoulder muscles.

Steps:

1. Sit upright in a chair with your feet firmly planted on the floor. This stable base supports proper posture and alignment throughout the exercise.

2. Inhale deeply, and with intention, lift your shoulders towards your ears. This upward movement should be controlled, engaging the muscles without straining them.

3. As you exhale, consciously release your shoulders back down. This downward motion encourages relaxation and the release of any built-up tension.

4. Repeat the shrugging motion 5-10 times, focusing on smooth, deliberate movements. Each shrug should contribute to a greater sense of ease in your shoulders and neck.

Targeted Areas:
Spine and abdominal muscles.

Benefits:

An effective way to enhance spinal mobility, alleviate back stiffness, and support digestive health.

Safety Precautions:

- Twist gently, avoiding any forceful movements.

- If you have a spine condition, consult a healthcare professional first.

Steps:

1. Begin by sitting upright in a chair, ensuring your feet are flat on the ground. This position helps maintain balance and proper spinal alignment during the twist.

2. Place your right hand on your left knee and your left hand behind you on the chair. These hand placements provide stability and support for the twist.

3. Inhale deeply to prepare. As you exhale, gently twist your torso to the left. This movement should originate from the base of your spine, ensuring a gentle and effective stretch.

4. Hold the twist for a few breaths, allowing your body to relax into the position. This holding phase aids in deepening the stretch while supporting spinal health and digestion.

5. Slowly return to the center before repeating the exercise on the opposite side. This ensures balanced mobility and flexibility on both sides of the body.

Targeted Areas:
Lower and upper back.

Benefits:

Strengthens back muscles, enhancing posture, and increasing spinal flexibility.

Safety Precautions:

- Do not overextend your back.
- Move into the position slowly and smoothly.

Steps:

1. Sit at the edge of a stable chair with your feet firmly planted on the ground. This starting position ensures a solid foundation for the exercise.

2. Place your hands on your thighs for support. This helps maintain balance and alignment as you move through the spinal extension.

3. Inhale deeply and gently begin to arch your back. Push your chest forward and draw your shoulders back, engaging the muscles along your spine.

4. Hold this arched position for a few seconds, allowing your back muscles to stretch and strengthen. Be mindful not to overextend; the movement should be comfortable and controlled.

5. Exhale slowly and return to your starting position, feeling the length and relaxation in your spine.

6. Repeat the exercise 5-7 times, focusing on smooth, deliberate movements. Each repetition will contribute to a greater sense of strength and flexibility in your back.

Targeted Areas:

Lateral muscles, obliques, and ribcage.

Benefits:

Improves flexibility and can help reduce stiffness in the sides and back, contributing to overall comfort and mobility.

Safety Precautions:

- Stretch only as far as comfortable.

- Avoid this exercise if you have severe rib or spine issues.

Steps:

1. Start by sitting upright in a chair with your feet flat on the ground, establishing a stable and comfortable base.

2. Inhale and raise your right arm overhead, ensuring your posture remains straight and aligned.

3. As you exhale, gently lean to the left. This movement stretches the right side of your body, from the ribcage to the obliques. Move into the stretch only as far as feels comfortable, avoiding any strain.

4. Hold the position for a few breaths, allowing the stretch to deepen with each exhale. This not only enhances the stretch but also aids in relaxation.

5. Slowly return to the center and lower your arm. Then, repeat the stretch on the left side, raising your left arm and leaning to the right.

SEATED WARRIOR II ARMS

Targeted Areas:
Arms, shoulders, and upper back.

Benefits:

A fantastic way to fortify and stretch arms and shoulders while also sharpening your focus.

Safety Precautions:

• Keep the shoulder blades down and back to avoid tension.

Steps:

1. Begin by sitting upright in a chair, ensuring your feet are flat on the ground. This stable base aids in maintaining proper posture throughout the exercise.

2. Stretch your arms out to either side, reaching them to shoulder height with your palms facing down. This action engages the muscles in your arms and shoulders, promoting strength and flexibility.

3. Turn your head to gaze over your right hand, extending the stretch and enhancing your focus. This not only helps in stretching the neck muscles but also aids in concentration and mental clarity.

4. Hold this position for several deep breaths, encouraging a deeper engagement with each exhale. Ensure your shoulder blades are drawn down and back to prevent any unnecessary tension in your neck and shoulders.

5. Gently bring your gaze back to the center before turning to look over your left hand, effectively repeating the pose on this side. This ensures a balanced stretch and strength enhancement across both sides of your body.

"Explore Micro-Movements"

In each pose, experiment with subtle shifts—tilting your pelvis, adjusting your shoulder blades, or turning your palms. These micro-movements can deepen the pose's effect and increase body awareness.

POSES FOR MOBILITY

Targeted Areas:

Arms and shoulders.

Benefits:

Improve shoulder mobility, increase upper body strength, and enhance circulation.

Safety Precautions:

• Keep your movements slow and controlled to avoid any strain on your shoulders.

• If you experience any pain or discomfort, reduce the size of your circles or take a break.

Steps:

1. Begin by sitting upright in a chair, with your feet flat on the ground.

2. Extend your arms out to the sides at shoulder height, keeping them straight. Ensure your palms are facing down to start, positioning your body in a T-shape.

3. Start making small circles with your arms, moving them in a forward motion. Focus on keeping the circles controlled and your arms level with your shoulders.

4. Gradually increase the size of the circles as you become more comfortable, ensuring you maintain control and do not strain your shoulder muscles.

5. After 15 seconds or when you're ready, reverse the direction of your circles, moving your arms in a backward motion. This change helps to engage different muscles.

6. Continue performing the arm circles for a total of 30 seconds to 1 minute, alternating between forward and backward motions.

CHAIR CAT-COW STRETCH

Targeted Areas:
Spine, neck, and shoulders.

Benefits:

This gentle movement helps increase spine flexibility and relieve tension in the back and neck. It can also aid in improving posture and breathing.

Safety Precautions:

- Move slowly and gently to avoid any strain.
- If you have severe back pain or a spinal injury, consult with a healthcare provider before attempting this exercise.

Steps:

1. Sit upright towards the front edge of a stable chair, placing your feet flat on the floor, hip-width apart. Place your hands on your knees or thighs for support.

2. Begin with the Cow pose: Inhale, arch your back, and tilt your pelvis back, sticking your buttocks out slightly. Lift your chest and chin upwards, gazing slightly forward or up, and pull your shoulders back. This position encourages a gentle arch in your lower back, opening the chest and stretching the front of your torso.

3. Transition to the Cat pose: Exhale, round your spine, and tilt your pelvis forward, tucking your tailbone under. Draw your chin towards your chest, gaze down at your navel, and push your mid-back towards the chair back. This movement stretches the back of your spine and releases tension in your neck and shoulders.

4. Continue to flow smoothly between the Cow and Cat poses, following the rhythm of your breath: Inhale as you move into Cow pose, and exhale as you transition into Cat pose.

5. Repeat this sequence for several breath cycles (typically 5-10), focusing on the sensation of movement along your spine and the relaxation of tension with each transition.

"Engage Your Senses"

Integrate aromatherapy or calming sounds into your practice environment. A drop of lavender oil on your wrists or calming nature sounds can deepen relaxation and enhance the sensory experience of your practice.

SEATED SHOULDER ROLLS

Targeted Areas:
Shoulders, neck, and upper back

Benefits:

This simple yet effective exercise is designed to release tension in the shoulders and neck, improve mobility, and enhance posture.

Safety Precautions:

- Perform the movements slowly and gently to avoid any strain.

- Keep your spine straight and aligned to prevent slouching during the exercise.

- Breathe naturally, coordinating your breath with the movement for maximum relaxation.

Steps:

1. Begin sitting upright in a chair with your feet flat on the floor, hip-width apart. Place your hands on your thighs or let them hang by your sides.

2. Inhale deeply, and as you exhale, slowly lift your shoulders towards your ears.

3. Continue the movement by gently rolling your shoulders back, drawing your shoulder blades towards each other to open up the chest.

4. As you complete the backward roll, lower your shoulders, creating a circular motion.

5. Once your shoulders are in their lowest position, begin the next roll by lifting them towards your ears again, then forward, up, back, and down, reversing the direction.

6. Perform this circular motion slowly and smoothly for several repetitions, typically 5-10 times in each direction, focusing on the sensation of release and relaxation in your shoulder and neck area.

7. Pause for a moment after completing the rolls in both directions, taking a few deep breaths to settle into the relaxation and openness created by the exercise.

Targeted Areas:

Torso, hips and lower back.

Benefits:

A gentle yet effective exercise for seniors, aimed at increasing hip and lower back mobility and alleviating stiffness in these areas.

Safety Precautions:

• Ensure the chair is stable.

• Avoid this exercise if you have severe hip pain.

Steps:

1. Begin by sitting near the edge of a stable chair. Place your feet firmly on the floor, hip-width apart, establishing a strong foundation.

2. Rest your hands on your hips for added stability. This also helps in maintaining an upright posture throughout the exercise.

3. Initiate the movement by gently guiding your upper body in a circular motion to the right. Ensure the motion originates from the torso, engaging the muscles around the hip joint and lower back.

4. Continue the circular motion, moving your torso back, then to the left, and finally bringing them forward. This motion should be fluid and controlled, focusing on the range of motion that feels comfortable.

5. Complete five circles in this direction, then reverse the direction for another five circles. The reversal ensures balanced mobility & muscle engagement on both sides.

CHAIR ASSISTED LEG LIFTS

Targeted Areas:
Thighs and core.

Benefits:

Strengthen the thighs while also enhancing stability and balance.

Safety Precautions:

- Move slowly and control the movement.

- Do not overextend if you have knee problems.

Steps:

1. Begin by sitting upright in a stable chair, ensuring your feet are flat on the ground. This starting position promotes good posture and prepares your body for the exercise.

2. Grasp the sides of the chair lightly for support. This not only aids in maintaining balance during the exercise but also ensures safety and control.

3. Carefully extend one leg out in front of you, striving to keep it parallel to the floor. The goal is to activate the muscles in your thigh and core without straining them.

4. Hold this extended position for a few seconds, focusing on engaging the thigh muscles while keeping the rest of your body stable.

5. Gently lower the leg back to the starting position, controlling the movement to maximize the exercise's benefits.

6. Perform 5-10 repetitions with each leg, alternating to ensure balanced strength and flexibility in both legs.

Targeted Areas:

Spine and lower back.

Benefits:

An excellent exercise for focusing on stretching the spine and lower back. It not only eases tension in these areas but also aids in calming the mind.

Safety Precautions:

- Bend from your hips, not your waist.
- Avoid if you have severe lower back issues.

Steps:

1. Start by sitting upright on a secure chair. Keep your feet planted on the floor, ensuring they are parallel and hip-width apart for stability.

2. Inhale deeply and raise your arms overhead, bringing a gentle stretch to your upper body. This upward movement also aids in elongating the spine.

3. As you exhale, gradually hinge forward from your hips, not the waist. This distinction is crucial for targeting the right muscles and ensuring safety.

4. Extend your hands towards your feet or shins, depending on your comfort and flexibility. The key is to stretch without straining.

5. Hold for a few deep breaths, allowing the stretch to penetrate your spine and lower back. Focus on the sensation of release in your back with each exhale.

6. Slowly rise back to the sitting position, using your hands for support if necessary.

Poses for Flexibility and Balance

Benefits:

Aimed at strengthening the calf muscles and improving ankle stability. This exercise is crucial for maintaining mobility, balance, and support during daily activities.

Safety Precautions:

- Move slowly and avoid jerky movements.
- If you have ankle or calf injuries, proceed with caution.

Steps:

1. Start by sitting upright in a chair with your feet flat on the floor. Ensure your posture is straight, supporting overall alignment and balance.

2. Gradually raise your heels off the floor, shifting your weight onto the balls of your feet. This movement engages the calf muscles, promoting strength and stability.

3. Hold this raised position for a few seconds. This pause is key to maximizing muscle engagement and enhancing stability in the ankles.

4. Gently lower your heels back to the floor, controlling the movement to ensure smooth and steady strengthening.

5. Repeat the calf raise 10-15 times. This repetition range is optimal for building strength and endurance in the calf muscles and ankles.

CHAIR TREE

Targeted Areas:
Legs, ankles, and core.

Benefits:

A chair yoga pose that focuses on improving balance, strengthening the ankles and calves, and enhancing focus.

Safety Precautions:

•Avoid if you have severe knee or hip problems.

OPTIONAL

Steps:

1. Begin by sitting upright in a stable chair, with your feet firmly planted on the floor. This position ensures proper posture and balance from the start.

2. Carefully place your right foot on top of the left thigh, making sure to avoid resting it directly on the knee joint. For a less intense variation, rest your right foot on your left ankle instead.

3. Gently press your right knee towards the floor to open up the hip. This movement should be done gently to avoid strain, focusing on the stretch and opening of the hip.

4. Bring your hands together in a prayer position at your chest or, for an added challenge, raise them overhead, keeping your shoulders away from your ears. This adds an element of balance and focus to the pose.

5. Hold this position for 5-10 breaths, focusing on maintaining balance and stability. The breath will aid in concentration and steadiness.

6. After completing one side, gently release and switch sides, repeating the process with the left foot on the right thigh or ankle.

SEATED LEG STRETCHES

Benefits:

It enhances flexibility in the hamstrings and lower back, crucial for improving mobility and easing daily movements.

Safety Precautions:

- Do not overstretch; go only as far as comfortable.

- Avoid if you have severe sciatica.

Steps:

1. Start by sitting on the edge of a stable chair, ensuring your posture is upright. This initial position helps maintain balance and alignment for an effective stretch.

2. Fully extend one leg forward, resting the heel on the ground and toes pointing upwards. If you find it challenging, it's perfectly fine to keep a slight bend in the knee. This position targets the hamstring and calf of the extended leg.

3. Keep the other foot flat on the floor to support balance and stability.

4. Inhale deeply to prepare. As you exhale, gently lean forward from your hips towards the extended leg. This forward motion enhances the stretch in the hamstring and lower back. Move into the stretch only as far as comfortable, avoiding any strain.

5. Hold the position for a few breaths, allowing the stretch to deepen gently with each exhale. This not only aids in flexibility but also promotes relaxation.

6. After holding, gently return to the starting position and switch legs, repeating the stretch to ensure balanced flexibility on both sides.

Targeted Areas:
Spine, abdominal muscles, and back.

Benefits:

An effective exercise designed to enhance spinal mobility, relieve back stiffness, and support digestion and stress relief.

Safety Precautions:

- Twist gently, avoiding any forceful movements.
- If you have a spine condition, consult a healthcare professional first.

Steps:

1. Begin by sitting upright on a stable chair, with your feet flat on the floor.

2. Cross your left leg over your right, placing your left foot beside your right knee. This setup prepares your body for a deeper twist and stretch.

3. Place your right hand on your left knee and your left hand behind you on the chair. These hand placements aid in supporting the twist and ensuring stability.

4. Inhale deeply to prepare your body. As you exhale, gently twist your torso to the left, aiming to look over your left shoulder. This movement initiates the twist from your lower back, extending up through your spine to your neck.

5. Hold the position for a few breaths, allowing the twist to deepen gently with each exhale. Focus on feeling the stretch throughout your spine.

6. After holding, slowly return to the center before repeating the exercise on the opposite side. This ensures balanced flexibility and mobility in both directions.

SEATED KNEE LIFTS

Targeted Areas:
Thighs and hips.

Benefits:

Focuses on strengthening thigh muscles and improving hip mobility.

Safety Precautions:

- Lift the knee only as high as comfortable.
- Avoid if you have acute hip pain.

Steps:

1. Begin by sitting upright on a stable chair, ensuring your feet are flat on the ground. This starting posture helps maintain balance and alignment during the exercise.

2. Place your hands on your thighs or the sides of the chair for additional stability. This support is crucial for maintaining proper form throughout the movement.

3. Slowly lift one knee towards your chest, keeping the movement controlled and the other foot flat on the floor. This action engages the thigh muscles and encourages hip mobility.

4. Hold the lifted position for a few seconds, focusing on engaging your core and thigh muscles. This hold increases muscle strength and stability.

5. Gently lower the leg back to the starting position, ensuring the movement is smooth and controlled.

6. Alternate legs, performing 10-15 lifts per leg. This repetition ensures balanced strength and flexibility in both hips and thighs.

Targeted Areas:

Calves and feet.

Benefits:

Excellent exercise for those looking to enhance lower leg strength, boost circulation, and improve coordination.

Safety Precautions:

- Tap gently to avoid jarring your legs.
- Suitable for those with limited lower body mobility.

Steps:

1. Position yourself upright in a chair, ensuring your feet are placed flat on the ground. This posture ensures stability and alignment as you perform the toe taps.

2. Engage your leg muscles to lift your toes while keeping your heels firmly planted on the floor. This action begins the strengthening and circulation enhancement in the lower legs.

3. Gently tap your toes back down to the floor, creating a rhythmic motion. The tapping not only strengthens the muscles but also promotes coordination and agility in the feet and calves.

4. Continue this tapping motion for 20-30 seconds, maintaining a steady pace. Focus on the movement of lifting and lowering the toes, ensuring each tap is controlled and deliberate.

5. Throughout the exercise, keep your posture upright and your movements smooth to maximize the benefits and minimize any risk of strain.

POSES FOR WEIGHT LOSS

Targeted Areas:

Arms, especially biceps and triceps.

Benefits:

This exercise strengthens the arms and improves elbow joint mobility.

Safety Precautions:

- Move in a controlled manner.
- If you have elbow or shoulder pain, proceed cautiously.

Steps:

1. Sit upright on a chair, ensuring stability and proper posture. This initial position is key for alignment and effectiveness of the exercise.

2. With arms extended forward and elbows bent at a 90-degree angle, you're positioned to begin the strengthening movement.

3. Smoothly extend your arms straight, then bend the elbows to bring your fists towards your shoulders. This motion engages the arm muscles in a controlled manner.

4. Repeat this bending and extending action 10-15 times, focusing on a fluid movement to maximize muscle engagement and joint mobility.

5. The controlled pace helps in focusing on muscle strength and joint flexibility, making each repetition effective.

CHAIR SUN SALUTATION

Targeted Areas:
Full body, including spine, arms, and legs.

Benefits:

A comprehensive exercise that enhances overall flexibility, boosts energy, and improves breathing.

Safety Precautions:

- Move through each step smoothly and avoid overstretching.
- Be mindful of your breathing.

Steps:

1. Position yourself upright in a chair with your feet firmly planted on the ground, establishing a stable foundation.

2. Inhale deeply and raise your arms overhead, directing your gaze upwards, inviting energy and openness into your body.

3. Exhale and fold forward from the hips, extending your hands towards your feet. This forward bend encourages flexibility in the spine and legs.

4. Inhale and lift your torso halfway up, achieving a straight back. This movement helps to lengthen the spine and refresh the posture.

5. Exhale and fold forward again, deepening the stretch and promoting relaxation.

6. With another inhalation, rise up smoothly, stretching your arms overhead once more, embracing a full body stretch.

7. Exhale and bring your hands to your heart, centering your energy and focus as you conclude the sequence.

8. Repeat this sequence 3-5 times, flowing through each step with mindfulness and ease.

SEATED KNEE EXTENSIONS

Benefits:

Excellent way to strengthen thigh muscles and enhance knee joint mobility.

Safety Precautions:

- Extend your knee gently.
- Avoid if you have severe knee pain.

Steps:

1. Begin by sitting upright on a chair, ensuring your feet are firmly on the ground.

2. Extend one leg out in front of you, preparing for the lift. This action sets the stage for strengthening the muscles around your knee.

3. Slowly raise and lower the extended leg, maintaining a smooth and controlled movement. This precision helps in maximizing muscle engagement while protecting the knee joint.

4. Aim for 10-15 lifts, focusing on the quality of movement rather than speed. Each lift contributes to building strength in the thigh muscles and improving flexibility in the knee joint.

5. After completing the set, switch to the other leg to ensure balanced strengthening across both legs.

Targeted Areas:

Thighs, hips, and buttocks.

Benefits:

Excellent exercise for those looking to enhance lower leg strength, boost circulation, and improve coordination.

Safety Precautions:

• Squat only as low as comfortable.

Steps:

1. Begin by standing in front of a stable chair, ensuring it's securely positioned to support you if needed. Your feet should be hip-width apart, aligning your body for optimal movement.

2. Initiate the squat by slowly lowering your body, as if intending to sit down. This movement engages the muscles in your thighs, hips, and buttocks, building strength and flexibility.

3. Bend at the knees and hips, keeping your chest upright and core engaged. This posture ensures a safe, effective squat that targets the right areas without strain.

4. Before making contact with the chair, press through your heels to stand back up. This phase of the exercise challenges your balance and strength, enhancing stability.

5. Aim to complete 10-15 repetitions, maintaining a smooth, controlled motion throughout. Each squat should be performed with care, focusing on form and comfort.

SEATED JUMPING JACKS

Targeted Areas:
Full body, especially the arms and legs.

Benefits:

A low-impact alternative to traditional jumping jacks, perfect for seniors seeking to increase their heart rate, improve cardiovascular health, and boost coordination.

Safety Precautions:

- Move in a controlled manner.
- If you have joint issues, be cautious with the movements.

Steps:

1. Begin by sitting upright in a chair, legs together, and arms resting at your sides. Activate your lower abdominal muscles to reduce strain on your back. This starting position ensures stability and readiness for the movement.

2. With a smooth, coordinated motion, extend your legs simultaneously raising your arms above your head. This action mimics the dynamic motion of standing jumping jacks, engaging multiple muscle groups.

3. Carefully return to the starting position, maintaining control and balance throughout the movement. This return phase is crucial for coordinating the exercise and ensuring safety.

4. Aim for 10-20 repetitions, adjusting the number based on your comfort and fitness level. Each repetition should be performed with intention, focusing on controlled movements to maximize benefits while minimizing the risk of strain.

Targeted Areas:

Core, lower abdominals, and hip flexors.

Benefits:

Focuses on strengthening the core and lower abdominal muscles while also improving leg mobility.

Safety Precautions:

- Move in a controlled manner to prevent lower back strain.
- Suitable for those with a moderate level of abdominal strength.

Steps:

1. Begin by sitting on the edge of a chair. This position allows you to maintain balance and ensures the effectiveness of the exercise. Lean slightly back, but ensure your spine remains aligned to avoid any strain on your back.

2. Hold onto the sides of the chair for support. This grip will help you maintain your balance and position as you perform the flutter kicks.

3. Extend your legs in front of you, raising them slightly off the floor. Keep your legs straight, engaging your core muscles to support the movement.

4. Start to alternately lift each leg in a small, fluttering motion. This action should be controlled and steady, focusing on engaging the lower abdominals and hip flexors with each flutter.

5. Continue the flutter kicks for 30 seconds to 1 minute, depending on your comfort and ability. The goal is to maintain a steady pace and controlled movement throughout the exercise to maximize the benefits while minimizing the risk of strain.

POSES FOR HEART HEALTH AND STAMINA

Targeted Areas:

Chest, shoulders, and upper back.

Benefits:

Designed to improve posture, open up the chest, and alleviate respiratory discomfort. This exercise promotes a more upright posture and facilitates easier breathing.

Safety Precautions:

- Avoid overextending your back.
- If you have lower back issues, proceed cautiously.

Steps:

1. Begin by sitting upright in a chair with your feet firmly planted on the floor. This stable position ensures proper alignment and support throughout the exercise.

2. Clasp your hands behind your back. This action prepares your upper body for the stretch and helps in engaging the correct muscles.

3. Inhale deeply, and as you exhale, gently pull your clasped hands downwards. Simultaneously, open your chest and lift your gaze slightly upwards. This movement stretches the chest and shoulders, encouraging a natural opening of the upper body.

4. Hold this position for several breaths, allowing the stretch to deepen with each exhale. The focus should be on maintaining a gentle stretch that opens the chest without straining the back.

5. Carefully release the stretch and relax. The controlled return to a relaxed state helps in maximizing the benefits of the stretch while ensuring safety.

SEATED EAGLE ARMS

Targeted Areas:
Shoulders, upper back, and arms.

Benefits:

Designed to increase shoulder mobility, stretch the upper back, and relieve tension in the neck and shoulders.

Safety Precautions:

• Do not strain your shoulders; keep the movement gentle.

• Avoid if you have severe shoulder pain.

Steps:

1. Begin by sitting upright, ensuring your feet are firmly planted on the ground. This position stabilizes your base, allowing for a focused stretch in the upper body.

2. Extend your arms straight in front of you at shoulder height, preparing your muscles.

3. Cross your right arm over your left, bend your elbows and twist your forearms until your palms meet. This alignment targets the stretch in the shoulders and upper back.

4. Gently lift your elbows while consciously lowering your shoulders away from your ears. This deepens the stretch, enhancing the mobility and flexibility of the shoulder joints.

5. Hold this position for several breaths, focusing on the stretch and release of tension in the upper body.

6. Slowly unwind your arms and repeat the exercise on the opposite side.

Targeted Areas:

Hips, thighs, and lower back.

Benefits:

It enhances hip mobility and leg flexibility while improving circulation.

Safety Precautions:

• Swing your leg gently to avoid strain.

• Ensure the chair is stable.

Steps:

1. Sit at the edge of a stable chair with your feet planted firmly on the floor. This starting position ensures a solid base and prepares your body for movement.

2. Grasp the sides of the chair with both hands for stability. This support is crucial for maintaining balance during the exercise.

3. Extend one leg forward, keeping it as straight as comfortable. This extension prepares your leg for the swinging motion.

4. Gently swing the extended leg from side to side, allowing it to cross in front of your stationary leg. This movement should be controlled and within a comfortable range to avoid strain.

5. Continue the swinging motion for 10-15 repetitions, focusing on smooth, fluid movements to maximize the stretch and mobility benefits.

6. After completing the swings with one leg, pause for a moment to reset, then switch to the other leg, repeating the swinging motion for 10-15 repetitions.

SEATED SPHINX POSE

Targeted Areas:
Spine, chest, and shoulders.

Benefits:

Designed for seniors to strengthen the spine, open the chest and shoulders, and potentially alleviate lower back pain. It supports improved posture and respiratory function.

Safety Precautions:

- Keep your movements gentle and avoid straining your lower back.
- If you have severe back issues, consult a healthcare professional first.

Steps:

1. Position yourself at the front edge of a chair, ensuring your feet are planted firmly on the ground, shoulder-width apart.

2. Initiate the movement by bending forward from your hips, keeping your spine straight to maintain its natural curvature.

3. Slide your hands down your thighs while gently lowering your elbows to rest them on your thighs, transitioning smoothly into the pose.

4. Adjust your position so your elbows are directly beneath your shoulders, forming a 90-degree angle with your arms. This alignment replicates the traditional Sphinx Pose while seated, focusing on spinal integrity and shoulder openness.

5. Slightly lift your chest, creating a gentle arch in your back. This movement emphasizes spinal extension and chest opening, enhancing the stretch.

6. Extend your neck forward, keeping it in line with your spine, to ensure a comprehensive stretch without straining.

7. Hold this position for 5 breaths, focusing on deep, steady inhalations and exhalations to support relaxation and effectiveness of the pose.

8. To conclude, gently raise your torso back to the starting position. Aim for up to 3 repetitions, each time focusing on maintaining smooth movements and proper alignment.

Seated Upward Arm Stretch

Benefits:

Designed to stretch the arms and sides, enhance posture, and alleviate mild back discomfort.

Safety Precautions:

- Stretch within your comfortable range.
- Avoid if you have severe shoulder pain.

OPTIONAL

Steps:

1. Begin by sitting upright on a stable chair, feet grounded on the floor. This posture forms the foundation for a safe and effective stretch.

2. As you inhale, extend both arms overhead, ensuring your shoulders remain down and away from your ears to maintain relaxation in the neck.

3. For an added stretch, interlace your fingers and gently turn your palms upward, towards the ceiling. This intensifies the stretch along arms and sides of the torso.

4. Reach upwards as you keep your spine elongated, imagining each vertebra stretching away from the next. This action not only stretches the arms and sides but also encourages a tall, healthy posture.

5. Hold this uplifted position for a few deep breaths, allowing the stretch to deepen naturally with each exhale.

6. Gently lower your arms back to your sides as you exhale, feeling the release throughout your shoulders and arms.

Targeted Areas:

Shoulders, upper back, chest, and core muscles.

Benefits:

To enhance hip mobility and leg flexibility while improving circulation.

Safety Precautions:

• Move within a comfortable range to avoid shoulder discomfort.

• Keep your spine neutral to prevent undue strain on the back.

Steps:

1. Sit upright on a chair with feet flat on the ground, shoulder-width apart, providing a stable and supportive base.

2. Raise both arms towards the ceiling while engaging your core to stabilize your shoulders and ribcage.

3. Gently tuck your chin to maintain alignment of your head with your spine, avoiding forward head posture.

4. Exhale and bend your elbows, lowering your arms until they are parallel to the floor, with palms facing forward. Draw your shoulder blades together and gently lift your chest, creating the cactus arm shape.

5. Inhale and extend your arms back towards the ceiling, keeping your core engaged for stability and support.

6. Perform this bending and straightening motion 3-5 times, focusing on the movement's smoothness and the sensation of stretching and strengthening.

BEGINNER 28-DAY CHAIR YOGA CHALLENGE

Our Beginner 28-Day Chair Yoga Challenge is specifically crafted for seniors seeking gentle, yet effective strategies to increase flexibility and their range of motion, as well as help them manage pain such as arthritis pain. Engaging in these exercises over the next 28 days will gradually build strength without straining your muscles and enhance your balance to minimize the risks of falls. I have ensured these exercises are tailored to support the unique needs of seniors over 60. This specialized program will also promote relaxation, reduce stress, improve your mood, and foster greater independence in daily tasks.

This program will start off with very basic poses to help get you accustomed to chair yoga. Over the next few days and weeks, they will progress and you will feel yourself become more confident. Remember this is a process not an immediate change; some of you will feel the immediate benefits from chair yoga after your first week, and some of you will take the full 28 days to start feeling its positive effects. No matter what, I encourage you to stick with it and reach out for help, encouragement, or advice whenever you feel you need it. My email is jcharrisonbooks@gmail.com

To start, choose your program:

The Structured Daily Plan (page 91). Our structured daily program will hold your hand over the next 28 days and tell you exactly which exercise you should complete each day.

Or The Flexible Plan (page 103) This plan allows you to choose which exercises you would like to complete each day and gives you the freedom to change or repeat your favorite.

Instructions:

Here are the steps to get started with your chair yoga practice:

1. **Begin each day with a breathing exercise.** This will help to center your mind and prepare your body for the chair yoga session. Found on page 35

2. **Follow the sequence of poses as outlined for each day.** For Week 1, hold each pose for 30 seconds. Increase this to 40 seconds in Week 2, 45 seconds in Week 3, and 50 seconds in Week 4.

3. **Take a short pause of 15 seconds between each exercise or pose.** Use this time to breathe normally and prepare for the next pose.

4. **Remember to go at your own pace.** It's important to listen to your body and not push beyond comfort. If you experience any discomfort, modify the pose or skip it as needed.

5. **Begin with the goal of practicing these chair yoga workouts daily.** I know that you're busy, but I've found that this consistent approach helps students to establish a routine and maximize the benefits of the program.

   » However, it's important to listen to your body and be mindful of your energy levels and physical comfort.

   » If you find that daily practice is too demanding, or if you experience any discomfort, it's perfectly fine to adjust your schedule.

   » In such cases, aim to complete the workouts 4 to 5 times a week instead.

   » This adjustment ensures that you still maintain regular practice while giving your body adequate time to rest and recover.

I'm here to support you on your journey to a healthier, happier life. If you have any questions, concerns, or would like a few words of encouragement, please don't hesitate to reach out (jcharrisonbooks@gmail.com).

Ending Each Session:

When you're finished with your yoga practice, take a few moments to meditate. This will help you to calm your mind and body and to integrate the benefits of your practice.

» Sit in a comfortable position in your chair. Close your eyes and take a few deep breaths. Focus on your breath, and let go of any thoughts or worries that come to mind.

» After a few minutes, you may want to try a simple meditation technique, such as focusing on a mantra or visualization. Or, you can simply sit quietly and enjoy the feeling of relaxation. For the meditation chapter, see page 239.

» When you're ready, open your eyes and slowly come back to the present moment. Take a few moments to appreciate the sense of relaxation and well-being that you've created.

My students who have gone through this program often tell me that "the key to success in this program is consistency and self-awareness." Adapt the practice to fit your needs and enjoy the journey of gentle mobility and improved well-being.

Breathing Exercise: Diaphragmatic Breathing (3 minutes) p. 36

Wrist & Ankle Rotation	Shoulder Rolls	Cat-Cow Stretch	Forward Bend
30s (p. 43)	30s (p. 62)	30s (p. 60)	30s (p. 65)

Breathing Exercise: Box Breathing (3 minutes) p. 42

Gentle Twists	Neck Roll and Stretch	Spinal Twist	Spinal Extension
30s (p. 44)	30s (p. 51)	30s (p. 71)	30s (p. 54)

Breathing Exercise: Alternate Nostril Breathing (3 minutes) p. 39

Shoulder Stretch	Arm Circles	Leg Stretches	Leg Lifts
30s (p. 45)	30s (p. 59)	30s (p. 70)	30s (p. 64)

Breathing Exercise: Ocean Breath (3 minutes) p. 38

Toe and Heel Lifts	Chair Tree	Knee Lifts	Calf Raises
30s (p. 46)	30s (p. 68)	30s (p. 72)	30s (p. 67)

DAY 5: UPPER BODY MOBILITY

Breathing Exercise: Cooling Breath (3 minutes) p. 41

Seated Neck Rolls	Shoulder Shrugs	Eagle Arms	Elbow Bends
30s (p. 47)	30s (p. 52)	30s (p. 84)	30s (p. 75)

DAY 6: GENTLE CARDIO AND COORDINATION

Breathing Exercise: Three-Part Breath (3 minutes) p. 37

Gentle Backbend	Knee Lifts	Jumping Jacks	Sun Salutation
30s (p. 46)	30s (p. 72)	30s (p. 80)	1 time (p. 76)

Breathing Exercise: Three-Part Breath (3 minutes) p. 37

Side Neck Stretch	Review and practice poses from Days 1-6.
	Choose one pose from each day.
30s (p. 45)	30s each.

Breathing Exercise: Lion's Breath (3 minutes) p. 40

Wrist & Ankle Rotation	Torso Circles	Leg Stretches	Leg Lifts	Calf Raises
40s (p. 43)	40s (p. 63)	40s (p. 70)	40s (p. 64)	40s (p. 67)

Breathing Exercise: Box Breathing (3 minutes) p. 42

Gentle Twists	Shoulder Shrugs	Warrior II Arms	Elbow Bends	Upward Arm
40s (p. 44)	40s (p. 52)	40s (p. 56)	40s (p. 75)	40s (p. 88)

Breathing Exercise: Alternate Nostril Breathing (3 minutes) p. 39

Seated Neck Rolls	Cat-Cow Stretch	Spinal Twist	Spinal Ext.	Torso Twists
40s (p. 47)	40s (p. 60)	40s (p. 71)	40s (p. 54)	40s (p. 53)

DAY 11: BALANCE AND STABILITY

Breathing Exercise: Ocean Breath (3 minutes) p. 38

Side Neck Stretch	Chair Tree	Knee Lifts	Warrior II Arms	Leg Swings
40s (p. 45)	40s (p. 68)	40s (p. 72)	40s (p. 56)	40s (p. 85)

DAY 12: CARDIOVASCULAR FOCUS

Breathing Exercise: Lion's Breath (3 minutes) p. 40

Gentle Backbend	Jumping Jacks	Sun Salutation	Knee Ext.	Forward Bend
40s (p. 46)	40s (p. 80)	1-2 times (p. 76)	40s (p. 78)	40s (p. 65)

Breathing Exercise: Three-Part Breath (3 minutes) p. 37

Shoulder Stretch	Neck Roll & Stretch	Side Stretch	Torso Circles	Cactus Arms
40s (p. 45)	40s (p. 51)	40s (p. 55)	40s (p. 63)	40s (p. 89)

Breathing Exercise: Diaphragmatic Breathing (3 minutes) p. 36

Wrist & Ankle Rotation	Arm Circles	Spinal Twist	Elbow Bends	Forward Bend
40s (p. 43)	40s (p. 59)	40s (p. 71)	40s (p. 75)	40s (p. 65)

Breathing Exercise: Box Breathing (3 minutes) p. 42

Gentle Backbend	Torso Circles	Flutter Kicks	Knee Ext.	Toe Taps
45s (p. 46)	45s (p. 63)	45s (p. 81)	45s (p. 78)	45s (p. 73)

Day 16: Upper Body

Breathing Exercise: Alternate Nostril Breathing (3 minutes) p. 39

Seated Neck Rolls	Shoulder Shrugs	Eagle Arms	Upward Arm	Chest Opener
45s (p. 47)	45s (p. 52)	45s (p. 84)	45s (p. 88)	45s (p. 83)

Day 17: Spinal Mobility

Breathing Exercise: Ocean Breath (3 minutes) p. 38

Shoulder Stretch	Sphinx Pose	Warrior II Arms	Torso Twists	Side Stretch
45s (p. 45)	45s (p. 86)	45s (p. 56)	45s (p. 53)	45s (p. 55)

Day 18: Balance and Stability

Breathing Exercise: Lion's Breath (3 minutes) p. 40

Toe and Heel Lifts	Chair Tree	Knee Lifts	Leg Swings	Flutter Kicks
45s (p. 46)	45s (p. 68)	45s (p. 72)	45s (p. 85)	45s (p. 81)

Breathing Exercise: Cooling Breath (3 minutes) p. 41

Gentle Twists	Jumping Jacks	Sun Salutation	Knee Ext.	Neck Roll & Stretch
45s (p. 44)	45s (p. 80)	1-2 times (p. 76)	45s (p. 78)	45s (p. 51)

Breathing Exercise: Three-Part Breath (3 minutes) p. 37

Wrist & Ankle Rotation	Forward Bend	Spinal Twist	Torso Circles	Shoulder Rolls
45s (p. 43)	45s (p. 65)	45s (p. 71)	45s (p. 63)	45s (p. 62)

Breathing Exercise: Diaphragmatic Breathing (3 minutes) p. 36

Gentle Twists	Leg Stretches	Squats	Cactus Arms	Elbow Bends
45s (p. 44)	45s (p. 70)	45s (p. 79)	45s (p. 89)	45s (p. 75)

Breathing Exercise: Box Breathing (3 minutes) p. 42

Toe and Heel Lifts	Torso Circles	Leg Stretches	Leg Lifts	Toe Taps
50s (p. 46)	50s (p. 63)	50s (p. 70)	50s (p. 64)	50s (p. 73)

Breathing Exercise: Alternate Nostril Breathing (3 minutes) p. 39

Gentle Backbend	Shoulder Shrugs	Eagle Arms	Upward Arm	Warrior II Arms
50s (p. 46)	50s (p. 52)	50s (p. 84)	50s (p. 88)	50s (p. 56)

Breathing Exercise: Ocean Breath (3 minutes) p. 38

Seated Neck Rolls	Cat-Cow Stretch	Sphinx Pose	Torso Twists	Side Stretch
50s (p. 47)	50s (p. 60)	50s (p. 86)	50s (p. 53)	50s (p. 55)

Breathing Exercise: Lion's Breath (3 minutes) p. 40

Gentle Backbend	Chair Tree	Knee Lifts	Leg Swings	Toe Taps
50s (p. 46)	50s (p. 68)	50s (p. 72)	50s (p. 85)	50s (p. 73)

Breathing Exercise: Cooling Breath (3 minutes) p. 41

Shoulder Stretch	Jumping Jacks	Sun Salutation	Knee Ext.	Arm Circles
50s (p. 45)	50s (p. 80)	2-3 times (p. 76)	50s (p. 78)	50s (p. 59)

Breathing Exercise: Three-Part Breath (3 minutes) p. 37

Side Neck Stretch	Forward Bend	Spinal Twist	Torso Circles	Upward Arm
50s (p. 45)	50s (p. 65)	50s (p. 71)	50s (p. 63)	50s (p. 88)

Diaphragmatic Breathing		Warm-up	Review and practice	Closing
		Choose two of your favorite warm-ups to revisit	Choose your favorite poses to revisit	Relaxation and reflection session
3 minutes (p. 36)		50s each.	50s each.	

PRO TIP

"Focus on the Feet"

Even though you're seated, your feet play a crucial role. Press them firmly into the ground during poses to increase your sense of grounding and stability. This connection can enhance your overall posture and balance in seated positions.

Week-by-Week Guide

Welcome to the Flex Plan, here is how to get the most from this program over the next 28 days.

Getting Started:

» **Breathing and Warm-Up:** Before you begin, choose 1 breathing and 1 warm-up exercise, from Chapter Three (page 35), to start each day.

» **Choose Your Poses:** Each day, pick 3 or 4 poses that feel comfortable and enjoyable.

» **Flexibility in Your Routine:** Feel free to vary your poses daily. Adjust the duration to suit your energy levels and comfort.

» **Proceed at Your Pace:** Once your poses are selected, you're ready to continue with the program at a pace that feels right for you.

Remember: This journey is all about your wellness and flexibility, tailored to your unique needs and preferences. Let's take this step together, embracing health and joy at every turn!

Week 1: Introduction and Basic Mobility

» Duration per Pose: 20 - 30 seconds.

» Daily Session Length: Start with 5 minutes, gradually increase as comfortable.

» Focus: Gentle stretches and movements for neck, shoulders, and arms. Basic leg and ankle movements for circulation.

» Suggested Poses: Seated neck rolls, shoulder shrugs, wrist and ankle rotations.

» Breathing Exercises: Start and end with 1 minute of deep, mindful breathing.

Week 2: Strengthening and Flexibility

» Duration per Pose: 40 seconds.

» Daily Session Length: Aim for 7-10 minutes.

» Focus: Incorporate gentle core strengthening exercises and leg stretches. Begin introducing balance-focused poses with chair support.

» Suggested Poses: Seated cat-cow, seated knee extensions, and seated calf raises.

» Breathing Exercises: Diaphragmatic breathing before and after the session.

Week 3: Enhanced Balance and Coordination

» Duration per Pose: 45 seconds.

» Daily Session Length: Maintain at 10 minutes.

» Focus: Introduce more dynamic movements for coordination. Continue with balance poses, adding mild twists for flexibility.

» Suggested Poses: Seated twist for spine health, seated toe taps for coordination, and chair tree.

» Breathing Exercises: Alternate nostril breathing for focus and balance.

Week 4: Advanced Integration and Relaxation

» Duration per Pose: 50 seconds.

» Daily Session Length: Extend to 12-15 minutes.

» Focus: Combine strength, balance, and flexibility poses from previous weeks. Introduce advanced modifications for those who are comfortable.

» Suggested Poses: Full sequence combining all learned poses, with more advanced options as appropriate.

» Breathing Exercises: Ujjayi breath (ocean breath) to enhance concentration and relaxation.

Make a Difference with Your Review

"Kindness, like a boomerang, always returns." – Unknown

Did you know that the kindest folks are often the happiest? It's true! When we do something nice for someone else, without thinking about what we'll get in return, we're sprinkling a little magic into their lives and ours. So, how about we sprinkle some of that magic together?

I've got a little favor to ask of you...

Imagine being able to help someone just like you, someone who once felt a bit unsure about starting something new, like chair yoga. Remember what it was like wanting to feel better, move easier, and enjoy life more, but not knowing where to start?

Our goal is to make 10-Min Chair Yoga For Seniors something everyone can enjoy and benefit from. Every move, every stretch, every breath we take in this book is aimed at making life a bit brighter and better. But, to spread this joy and health far and wide, we need your help.

Believe it or not, your opinion is super powerful. When someone is thinking about trying chair yoga, they look for what others have to say about it. So, here's my big ask on behalf of a friend you haven't met yet:

Would you share a few kind words about this book in a review?

It's a simple act that costs nothing and takes just a moment, but it could make a world of difference to someone looking for a sign to start their journey towards a more joyful and active life. Your review could help...

...another grandparent play freely with their grandkids.

...someone regain confidence in moving around their home.

...bring a smile to someone's face as they discover what they can achieve.

...inspire someone to start their journey to wellness.

To spread a little kindness and make a big impact, all you need to do is leave a review. **It's easy:** Simply go to the link (https://geni.us/ChairYogaBook) or scan the QR code below to share your thoughts or go to your orders on Amazon:

If the thought of helping someone out there warms your heart, then you're exactly the kind of person I wrote this book for. Welcome to our community of kindness warriors. You're one of us now.

I'm thrilled to be on this journey with you, helping you discover easier movements and brighter days through chair yoga. I can't wait for you to experience the joy and freedom waiting for you in the pages ahead.

Thank you from the bottom of my heart. Let's get back to our yoga adventure.

Your biggest cheerleader, *J.C. Harrison*

PS - Remember, sharing is caring! If you believe this book could help another soul dance through their day a little easier, why not share it with them? It's a simple way to spread joy and kindness, making you and the recipient feel great.

Movement is a medicine for creating change in a person's physical, emotional, and mental states.

– Carol Welch

CHAPTER 5
INTERMEDIATE 28-DAY CHAIR YOGA CHALLENGE

In Chapter Five, you'll deepen your chair yoga practice with intermediate poses aimed at enhancing your physical abilities, directly impacting your everyday life. These exercises are designed to increase strength, flexibility, and balance, enabling activities that may have become challenging.

Imagine playing with your grandchildren with renewed energy, navigating stairs confidently, enjoying gardening with less strain, or taking pleasure in leisurely walks—all without the discomfort that once held you back.

In this chapter, we're going to take the next step together on your chair yoga journey. Moving from the basics we covered for beginners, we'll embrace the challenges and rewards of intermediate poses, specially tailored for seniors. As we progress, you'll notice not just improvements in your strength, balance and flexibility but in your daily life as well. This path we're on is deeply personal—it's about rediscovering the joy in movements and activities you love, and sharing those moments with the people who matter most. Let's continue to grow and explore, side by side.

The 28-Day Intermediate challenge can be found on page 152.

POSES FOR BETTER POSTURE

Targeted Areas:
Spine, chest, and shoulders.

Benefits:

A wonderful way to enhance your posture and fortify your legs, all while gently opening up the chest and shoulders.

Safety Precautions:

- Keep your back straight and avoid overextending.

- If you have balance issues, ensure the chair is stable.

Steps:

1. Begin by sitting at the edge of your chair, ensuring your feet are planted firmly on the ground and your arms rest comfortably at your sides.

2. With an inhalation, lift your arms above your head, allowing your palms to face each other, reaching towards the sky.

3. As you exhale, allow your back to gently arch, opening up your chest to the world and slightly tilting your head back, as if basking in the glow of the sun.

4. Engage the muscles in your thighs, feeling a connection through your legs, and elongate your spine as if a string is pulling you upwards.

5. Maintain this pose for a few deep breaths, feeling the stretch and openness.

6. On an exhale, slowly lower your arms back to your sides, returning to your starting position with a sense of renewal and strength.

SEATED FORWARD FOLD

Targeted Areas:
Hamstrings, spine, and lower back.

Benefits:

Gently stretching your spine and hamstrings.

Safety Precautions:

- Bend from your hips, not your waist. Start the movement at your hip joint, where your thigh meets your pelvis.

- Avoid if you have severe lower back issues.

Steps:

1. Begin by sitting upright, legs extended before you, with feet positioned hip-width apart. Let this be your foundation of stability and balance.

2. Inhale deeply, inviting length into your spine, envisioning each vertebra stretching towards the sky.

3. On your exhale, pivot gracefully from your hips (to bend from the hips push your hips back while keeping your spine long and chest open), folding forward as if reaching for a moment of tranquility. Extend your hands towards your feet, embodying the gentle embrace of calm.

4. Hold this forward embrace for several nurturing breaths, allowing tension to melt away with each exhale.

5. To conclude, slowly ascend back to an upright position, carrying with you the peace and stretch you've cultivated.

Targeted Areas:
Core, spine, chest, shoulders & hip flexors.

SEATED WARRIOR I WITH PRAYER HANDS

Benefits:

This variation strengthens the core, improves posture, and enhances spinal alignment.

Safety Precautions:

- Keep your front foot firmly planted on the ground to maintain balance.

- Avoid overextending the back; keep the movement in a comfortable range.

Steps:

1. Start by sitting upright towards the front edge of a stable chair, feet flat on the ground, turning your legs and body to the left side.

2. Extend one leg back, resting the foot on the ground, mimicking the stance of a traditional Warrior I but in a seated position. Ensure your front knee is directly over your ankle, forming a 90-degree angle.

3. Inhale and lace your hands in a prayer position at your heart center, engaging your core for stability. Draw your shoulders down away from your ears, engaging the core to support your spine.

4. Ensure your hips are facing forward, aligning your torso over your hips.

5. Hold the pose for several deep breaths, focusing on the stretch across your chest, shoulders, and the hip flexor of your extended leg.

6. To exit the pose, lower your arms and bring your extended leg back.

7. Repeat on the opposite side to ensure balance in the stretch.

CHAIR BUTTERFLY POSE

Targeted Areas:
Hips, groin, inner thighs, and pelvic floor.

Benefits:

Designed to gently open the hips, improve flexibility in the groin and inner thighs, and encourage pelvic floor relaxation.

Safety Precautions:

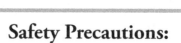

- Enter and exit the pose gently to avoid strain on the knees and hips.

- Adjust the height of the blocks according to your comfort level, choosing a height that allows you to maintain the pose without discomfort.

Steps:

1. Sit on a stable chair. If you don't have yoga blocks, consider alternatives like stacked books for firm support, firm pillows or cushions for softer support, sturdy boxes, folded blankets or towels for adjustable firmness, or robust shoe boxes. Place your chosen support on the floor in front of the chair, adjusting to a height that suits your flexibility—typically, the lowest or medium setting for most.

2. Sit towards the chair's front and bring the soles of your feet together, knees falling to the sides into the butterfly position. Place each foot on your chosen support.

3. Sit tall to lengthen your spine, bring your hands to your heart in a prayer pose or hold your knees for support and to avoid any strain.

4. Focus on relaxing into the stretch and stay in the position for several deep breaths. Use each exhale to potentially deepen the relaxation and stretch.

5. To release, carefully lift your knees, remove your feet from the supports, and bring legs together. Set aside the supports. take a few deep breaths to absorb the benefits.

Targeted Areas:

Chest, spine, and abdomen.

Benefits:

It's designed to strengthen and bring flexibility, enhancing your posture and breathing.

Safety Precautions:

- Avoid straining your lower back.

- If you have severe back issues, consult a healthcare professional first.

Steps:

1. Position yourself at the edge of your chair, ensuring your feet are solidly grounded.

2. Place your hands on either side of the chair, right beside your hips, ready to lift and support your body.

3. Press down into your hands, engage your core, and lift your chest toward the ceiling, allowing your back to gently arch as you direct your gaze upwards.

4. As you lift, draw your shoulders down and back, away from your ears, to open up the chest fully.

5. Maintain this uplifted posture for a few calming breaths, feeling the stretch across your chest and the strength in your spine.

6. Gently ease back into a neutral sitting position, carrying with you the openness and strength you've cultivated.

CHAIR WRIST STRETCH

Targeted Areas:
Wrists and forearms.

Benefits:

This stretch is aimed at increasing flexibility and reducing stiffness in the wrists and forearms.

Safety Precautions:

- Perform the stretch gently to avoid overextension or strain on the wrists.

- If you experience any pain or discomfort during the stretch, ease up on the intensity or discontinue the stretch.

- Keep your movements slow and controlled, especially when extending your arms and pressing your palms forward.

Steps:

1. Begin in a comfortable seated ensuring your spine is straight and shoulders are relaxed.

2. Gently interlace your fingers in front of you, ensuring a comfortable grip without squeezing too tightly.

3. With your fingers interlaced, flip your palms to face forward, away from your body. This action begins the process of engaging the wrists and forearms.

4. Carefully lift your arms to shoulder height, maintaining the interlaced fingers and forward-facing palms. Ensure your shoulders remain relaxed and down, away from your ears.

5. As you straighten your arms, press your palms forward, feeling a gentle stretch in the wrists and forearms. Ensure your arms are parallel to the floor, and you're pressing out as if against an invisible barrier.

6. Maintain this position for 5 deep breaths, focusing on the sensation of stretching and opening in the wrists and forearms. With each exhale, try to deepen the stretch slightly, without causing discomfort.

7. After holding for 5 breaths, gently release the interlace of your fingers and lower your arms back to your sides or lap. Shake out your hands and wrists gently if it feels comfortable.

POSES FOR MOBILITY

Targeted Areas:

Spine, abdominal muscles, and back.

Benefits:

The Chair Spinal Twist is a transformative exercise designed to increase spinal mobility, aid digestion, and alleviate back pain.

Safety Precautions:

- Twist gently and avoid straining.
- Consult a healthcare professional if you have severe back issues.

Steps:

1. Begin by sitting sideways on the chair, positioning yourself to face the left. This orientation prepares your body for the twist and ensures a full range of motion.

2. Grasp the back of the chair with both hands, establishing a firm grip that will aid in deepening the twist.

3. Take a deep inhalation to prepare your body. As you exhale, engage your core and twist your torso to the left, using your hands for gentle leverage. Look over your left shoulder to complete the twist, ensuring the movement extends throughout the spine.

4. Hold this position for a few breaths, allowing each exhalation to deepen the twist slightly, enhancing the stretch and its benefits on the spine and abdominal area.

5. To switch sides, gently release the twist and turn to face the right side of the chair. Repeat the twisting motion on this side to ensure a balanced, symmetrical stretch.

SEATED CHAIR PIGEON POSE

Targeted Areas:
Hips, glutes, and thighs.

Benefits:

A restorative stretch designed for those looking to open up the hips and glutes, stretch the thighs, and alleviate lower back pain.

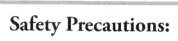

Safety Precautions:

- Be gentle to avoid stress on the knee.
- Avoid if you have severe hip or knee issues.

Steps:

1. Start by sitting upright in a chair, ensuring your feet are grounded on the floor for a stable base.

2. Gently place your right ankle on your left thigh, just above the knee, creating a figure-four shape. This position initiates the stretch in the hips and glutes.

3. Allow your right knee to relax, avoiding any forceful pressing. For a deeper stretch, gently apply pressure to your right knee with your hand, increasing the stretch in the outer hip and thigh.

4. Slowly lean forward, bending at the hips while keeping your spine straight and tall until you feel a stretch in your lower back.

5. Hold this position for several breaths, focusing on deep, steady breathing to facilitate relaxation and deepen the stretch.

6. Carefully release your leg and switch to the other side, repeating the pose to ensure balanced flexibility and relief in both hips.

Targeted Areas:

Legs, hips, and core.

Benefits:

Chair Eagle Legs is a seated adaptation of the classic yoga pose, tailored to improve balance, strengthen the thighs, and enhance focus.

Safety Precautions:

- Ensure stability and avoid over-twisting the legs.
- Not recommended if you have knee pain.

Steps:

1. Begin by sitting upright in a chair, ensuring your feet are planted firmly on the floor. This foundational stance aids in maintaining balance throughout the pose.

2. Carefully cross your left thigh over your right thigh, aiming to position it as high as comfortably possible. This crossing action initiates the engagement of the leg muscles and hips.

3. If you're able to, gently wrap your left foot around your right calf. This adds an extra element of balance and focus to the pose, challenging your stability further.

4. Actively squeeze your thighs together, maintaining this engagement for several breaths. This not only strengthens the leg muscles but also aids in core stability and focus.

5. After holding the pose, slowly unwind and prepare to repeat on the opposite side. This ensures a balanced workout, engaging both sides of the body equally.

SEATED DANCER POSE

Benefits:

A dynamic stretch, ideal for improving balance and concentration.

Safety Precautions:

- Be cautious to maintain balance.
- Avoid if you have knee or shoulder injuries.

Steps:

1. Start by sitting upright on the side of your chair, ensuring your feet are flat on the floor for a stable base.

2. Bend your left knee and grasp the outside of your left foot or ankle with your left hand. This action initiates the stretch and prepares your body for the pose.

3. Apply a gentle press with your foot against your hand while extending the leg slightly behind you. This extension opens up the thigh and shoulder, deepening the stretch.

4. For additional balance, extend your right arm forward or use the chair for stability. This helps maintain your balance and enhances the overall effectiveness of the pose.

5. Hold this position for several breaths, focusing on a steady, even breathing pattern to maximize the pose's benefits.

6. After holding, gently release and switch sides to ensure a balanced stretch across both sides of the body.

Targeted Areas:
Thighs, hips, and calves.

CHAIR HIGH LUNGE

Benefits:

Bolster your leg strength, elevate your balance, and stretch your hip flexors.

Safety Precautions:

- Ensure the chair is stable.
- Avoid this pose if you have severe knee or hip pain.

Steps:

1. Position yourself behind the chair, using the backrest as a support to ensure stability throughout the exercise.

2. Take a confident step backward with your left foot, bending your right knee to form a lunge. Your left leg should remain extended behind you, with the heel off the ground, creating a dynamic stretch.

3. Maintain an upright torso and ensure your hips are squared forward, aligning your body for maximum benefit.

4. Stay in this pose for a few deep breaths, feeling the strength in your legs and the stretch in your hips.

5. Gently release and switch legs, repeating the process to ensure balanced strength and flexibility across both sides of your body.

SEATED SIDE-TO-SIDE LEAN

Targeted Areas:
Side torso, obliques, and hips.

Benefits:

The Seated Side-to-Side Lean is an excellent exercise for gently stretching the side body, boosting flexibility, and improving lateral mobility.

Safety Precautions:

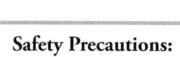

- Lean gently to avoid strain.
- Keep your buttocks firmly on the chair for stability.

Steps:

1. Start by sitting upright on a chair, with your feet planted firmly on the ground. This stable position ensures safety and effectiveness throughout the exercise.

2. Raise your arms overhead, interlocking your fingers with palms turned upward. This arm position helps maximize the stretch along the side body.

3. Take a deep breath in, and as you exhale, gently lean to the left, maintaining your extended arms. This movement stretches the right side of your torso, engaging the obliques and hips.

4. Inhale as you return to the center, preparing for the next stretch.

5. Exhale and lean to the right, stretching the left side of your body. This balanced approach ensures both sides of the torso are equally stretched and strengthened.

6. Continue this fluid, side-to-side motion for 5-10 repetitions, focusing on smooth, controlled movements. Each lean should be gentle to avoid any strain, with the buttocks remaining in contact with the chair for stability.

"Experiment with Breath Ratios"

Play with different breathing ratios (inhale to exhale) to find what soothes or energizes you. For example, try extending your exhales to promote relaxation or balance your inhale and exhale lengths for calming effects.

POSES FOR FLEXIBILITY AND BALANCE

Targeted Areas:

Legs, core, and ankles.

CHAIR-SUPPORTED TREE POSE

Benefits:

A gentle yet effective way to enhance your balance, strengthen your ankles, and sharpen your focus and concentration.

Safety Precautions:

- Keep your foot away from the knee joint to avoid pressure.
- Maintain a straight spine to prevent strain.

Steps:

1. Begin by standing beside your chair, using one hand to lightly hold onto the backrest for support. This touchpoint is your grounding, ensuring stability as you find your balance.

2. Carefully place your right foot against your inner left thigh or calf, making sure to avoid placing any pressure on your knee. This mindful placement is key to protecting your joints while engaging the muscles in your leg and core.

3. Elevate your right hand to a prayer position at your chest or reach it skyward, creating a line of energy that extends through your entire body. This gesture is not just about balance; it's a symbol of unity and focus.

4. Hold for several deep, calming breaths, allowing yourself to fully immerse in the moment. Feel the strength in your standing leg and the steadiness of your breath.

5. Gently release and switch sides, offering your body the same attention and care.

SEATED GODDESS POSE

Targeted Areas:
Thighs, hips, and groin.

Benefits:

This pose offers a gentle way to strengthen the thighs, open the hips, and improve lower body circulation while seated.

Safety Precautions:

- Adjust the width of your leg stance to avoid discomfort in the hips or knees.

- Keep your spine straight and avoid leaning forward to maintain balance and alignment.

- Engage your core throughout the pose for additional support.

Steps:

1. Sit comfortably towards the front of a stable chair, feet flat on the floor, and spine erect to maintain good posture.

2. Gently open your legs to each side, creating a V-shape with your legs. Adjust the width of your stance to a position that feels comfortable yet provides a gentle stretch in the inner thighs and groin area.

3. Turn your toes slightly outward, in alignment with the direction of your knees, to ensure a natural position that supports hip opening without strain.

4. Activate your abdominal muscles by drawing your navel towards your spine, supporting your upper body and promoting an upright posture.

5. For an added upper body stretch, raise your arms to shoulder height, bending the elbows so your forearms are vertical and palms face forward, resembling the cactus arm position. This can help open the chest and shoulders.

6. Maintain the Goddess Pose, breathing deeply for several breaths. Focus on the sensation of opening in the hips and thighs, and the strength being built in your posture.

7. To release, gently bring your legs back together, returning to the starting position. Lower your arms if they were raised.

8. Take a moment to sit with your feet planted and hands on your lap, breathing deeply to integrate the benefits of the pose.

SEATED DOWNWARD DOG POSE

Benefits:

It promotes improved circulation and offers relief from tension in the back and neck.

Safety Precautions:

- Maintain a neutral neck position.
- Adjust the intensity of the stretch to avoid discomfort, especially if you have back issues.

Steps:

1. Begin by sitting towards the front of your chair, creating an active and alert seated posture. Extend your legs straight in front of you, resting your heels on the floor, and flexing your toes towards you. Alternatively, if it feels more comfortable, bend your knees and place your feet flat on the floor.

2. With an inhale, extend your arms straight out in front of you or alongside your ears and fold forward slightly at your hips, not from the waist, and ensure your back is completely straight. Adjust the height of your arms to what feels most sustainable.

3. Actively draw your shoulder blades down and away from your ears, creating space and reducing tension in the neck and upper back.

4. Focus your gaze downward, toward your navel or at a fixed point on the ground between your legs. This helps maintain a neutral neck position & concentration.

5. Hold this position for several deep, even breaths. With each exhale, imagine releasing tension in the spine, shoulders, and hamstrings, deepening the stretch.

6. To exit the pose, gently raise your torso back up to an upright seated position on an inhale, lowering your arms to your sides or placing them on your lap.

Targeted Areas:
Hips, lower back, and ankles.

Benefits:

Gently promoting hip and lower back flexibility, enhancing circulation in the legs. Excellent for improving overall mobility.

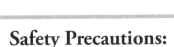

Safety Precautions:

- Ensure movements into and out of the pose are gentle to avoid straining the hips, knees, or ankles.

- Listen to your body and adjust the pose as necessary to avoid discomfort.

JNANA MUDRA

Steps:

1. Start seated comfortably towards the front of a stable chair, keeping your feet flat on the floor to start. Ensure your spine is erect, promoting an aligned posture.

2. Gently cross your ankles in front of you, allowing them to stay close to the floor. This position should create a mild, comfortable stretch in the hips.

3. Bring the backs of your hands to rest on your knees. Form Jnana Mudra by touching each thumb to its respective index finger, creating a circle, while keeping the rest of your fingers extended. This mudra promotes wisdom and concentration.

4. With your ankles crossed and hands in Jnana Mudra, sit tall and breathe deeply. Allow your shoulders to relax away from your ears, and close your eyes if comfortable to enhance the meditative aspect of the pose.

5. Stay in this pose for several deep breaths, focus on the sensation of relaxation and openness in your hips and lower back. Cultivate a sense of inner peace and calm.

6. To release, gently uncross your ankles and place your feet flat on the floor. Relax your hands and take a moment to notice any sensations in your body.

Seated Warrior II

Benefits:

It's a fantastic way to strengthen key muscle groups while also fostering mental resilience and focus.

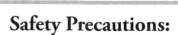

Safety Precautions:

- Ensure proper alignment to avoid strain.
- Avoid if you have hip or knee injuries.

Steps:

1. Begin by sitting on the edge of a chair, ensuring your spine is erect and your hands gently rest on your knees. Your feet should be flat on the floor, spaced apart at shoulder width for a stable foundation.

2. Open your left leg to the side, creating a 90-degree angle at the knee, with your foot firmly planted and toes pointing to the left. This movement begins the process of opening up the hips and strengthening the thigh muscles.

3. Extend your right leg back, straightening the knee, and place your foot flat on the ground with your toes pointing forward. This position stretches the hip flexors and calves, contributing to the overall strengthening of the lower body.

4. Elevate your arms to shoulder height, reaching them outward to the sides in a powerful stance. This not only strengthens the arms and shoulders but also helps in maintaining balance.

5. Turn your head to gaze towards your left hand, aligning your focus with your body's direction. Hold this posture for three to four deep breaths, feeling the strength and stability in your pose.

6. To release, gently turn your head back to the center, lower your arms, and bring your legs back to the initial position. This careful, controlled movement ensures a safe and effective practice.

7. Repeat the pose on the other side: Shift your right leg to the side this time, creating a 90-degree angle at the knee, and extend your left leg back. Turn your head to gaze towards your right hand. Hold for three to four breaths before returning to the starting position.

SEATED TRIANGLE POSE

Targeted Areas:
Spine, core, chest, hips, shoulders, inner thighs.

Benefits:

The Seated Triangle Pose offers a gentle yet effective way to stretch the sides of the body, improve spinal mobility, and enhance core strength.

Safety Precautions:

- Use the chair for support and move into the twist slowly.
- Avoid if you have severe balance or lower back issues.

Steps:

1. Begin by sitting on your chair, opening your knees as wide as it feels comfortable, ensuring a stable and grounded posture. Make sure your ankles are directly aligned under your knees, with your toes pointing in the same direction as your knees to maintain alignment and stability.

2. Inhale and extend your arms to a T position at shoulder height, preparing your body for the side stretch.

3. Push your hips slightly to the right side, and as you exhale, lean towards your left thigh, keeping your back straight and elongated to maximize the stretch along your right side.

4. Rest your left forearm gently on your left thigh for support, and extend your right arm upwards, reaching towards the sky. This position creates a dynamic stretch along the entire right side of your body, from your hips to your fingertips.

5. Turn your gaze upwards towards your right hand, encouraging a slight twist in your upper spine and deepening the stretch.

6. Hold the pose for a few breaths, focusing on the sensation of stretching and opening through your right side, maintaining a long and straight spine.

7. To exit the pose, inhale and gently bring your torso back to the center, arms extended to the sides at shoulder height.

8. Repeat the stretch on the opposite side, pushing your hips to the left and leaning towards your right thigh, to ensure a balanced stretch on both sides of your body.

POSES FOR WEIGHT LOSS

Targeted Areas:

Arms, shoulders, and core.

SEATED BOXING PUNCHES

Benefits:

A dynamic way to boost upper body strength, improve coordination, and enhance cardiovascular health.

Safety Precautions:

- Punch at a comfortable speed to avoid straining your shoulders or back.
- If you have joint pain in the arms or shoulders, proceed with caution.

Steps:

1. Begin by sitting at the edge of your chair, ensuring your feet are planted firmly on the ground. This position allows for maximum movement and stability.

2. Prepare your fists by clenching them and holding them up in front of your face, ready to engage in the exercise.

3. Alternately extend each arm forward in a punching motion, imagining you're hitting a boxing bag with each strike. This action not only strengthens the muscles but also improves coordination.

4. Maintain a rhythmic pace for 30 seconds to 1 minute, focusing on controlled movements to maximize the exercise's benefits without risking injury.

SEATED SUN SALUTATION FLOW II

Targeted Areas:
Spine, shoulders, arms, core muscles, hamstrings.

Benefits:

This sequence enhances spinal flexibility, boosts circulation, strengthens the core, and gently stretches the shoulders, arms, and hamstrings while reducing stress.

Safety Precautions:

• Move through the sequence at a pace that feels comfortable, avoiding any movements that cause discomfort.

• Keep movements smooth and controlled to prevent strain.

Steps:

1. Begin by sitting upright on your chair. Bring your hands to your heart, sitting tall and establishing a sense of grounding.

2. Open your arms to the sides and then move them all the way up overhead. As you reach the top, turn your hands so that your palms are facing forward.

3. Lower your arms to shoulder height, adopting the Cactus arms pose.

4. Lean forward halfway from your hips, pause, and then bring your hands to rest on your kneecaps. You have the option to keep your hands here or slowly slide them down your legs as you fold forward. Extend as far as feels comfortable, honoring your body's limits.

5. Lift halfway up, bringing your hands back to your knees for support.

6. Fold forward once more, and as you inhale, extend your right hand up, turning your head to look towards your right hand, while keeping your left hand on your left leg.

7. Exhale and lower your right hand, then inhale and switch, extending your left hand up to stretch the other side, turning your head to follow the movement.

8. Exhale, bring your left hand down, and as you inhale, lift your head and extend your arms to the side, reaching up, then bring your hands down to your heart.

9. Repeat this flow 3-5 times, moving with your breath and focusing on the fluidity and ease of the sequence.

CHAIR SQUAT TO STAND

Targeted Areas:
Thighs, hips, and glutes.

Benefits:

This exercise sharpens your balance and enhances functional mobility, making daily movements easier and more efficient.

Safety Precautions:

- Ensure the chair is stable.
- Avoid if you have severe knee or hip pain.

Steps:

1. Start seated in a chair with your feet planted firmly on the floor, shoulder-width apart, to ensure a strong foundation.

2. Initiate the movement by leaning slightly forward at the hips. This slight lean is crucial as it helps engage the correct muscles for standing.

3. Drive through your heels to stand up, using the strength in your legs and glutes to lift yourself. This part of the exercise is key for building power and stability in your lower body.

4. Reverse the motion by slowly sitting back down, controlling your descent to ensure it's smooth and measured. This controlled movement is just as important as standing up, as it engages your muscles differently and helps improve balance.

5. Aim to repeat this exercise 10-15 times, focusing on form and controlled movements. This repetition range offers a balanced approach to building strength and endurance.

Targeted Areas:

Spine, abdominal muscles, and arms.

CHAIR UPPER BODY TWISTS WITH ARMS EXTENDED

Benefits:

An excellent way to boost spinal mobility, core strength, and arm flexibility, contributing to an overall increase in upper body mobility and stability.

Safety Precautions:

- Twist gently to avoid straining the spine.
- Keep movements controlled and avoid overextending the arms.

Steps:

1. Begin by sitting upright on a chair with your feet flat on the ground, establishing a stable base.

2. Extend your arms to the sides at shoulder height, creating a T-shape with your body. This position prepares your upper body for the twisting motion.

3. Gently twist your upper body to the left, ensuring your arms remain extended. This movement engages your core and stretches the spine, promoting flexibility.

4. Slowly return to the center before twisting to the right. This alternating pattern ensures an even stretch and strengthening across your body.

5. Continue this sequence for 10-15 repetitions on each side, focusing on controlled movements to maximize benefits and minimize the risk of injury.

SUPPORTED CHAIR POSE

Targeted Areas:
Thighs, glutes, and lower back.

Benefits:

An excellent exercise for seniors looking to increase leg strength, enhance posture, and boost endurance and helps with better balance and supports daily activities.

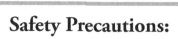

Safety Precautions:

• Keep your back straight and avoid leaning too far forward.

• Avoid if you have knee problems.

Steps:

1. Begin by standing in front of the back of your chair, placing your hands lightly on the top for initial support. Ensure your feet are shoulder-width apart and firmly on the ground for stability.

2. Take a deep breath in, engaging your core to keep your spine long and protected, start to bend your knees. Imagine you're about to sit down in a controlled descent.

3. As you lower your body, shift your grip to the sides of the chair backrest for added stability. Lower yourself to a comfortable depth, ideally until your thighs are about parallel to the floor, creating a stable base without straining.

4. Ensure your knees remain aligned with your toes, avoiding any inward or outward drifting. This alignment helps protect your joints. Maintain this squat position for five breaths, focusing on stability and the engagement of your leg muscles.

5. To rise, press down through your feet, using the strength of your legs and core to return to a standing position.

Benefits:

Aimed to fortify your obliques, boost lateral flexibility, and solidify core stability to help increase your balance and stability in daily life.

Safety Precautions:

- Use light weights and move slowly to avoid strain.
- If you have shoulder or back issues, do this exercise without weights.

Steps:

1. Position yourself upright in a chair with both feet planted firmly on the ground, creating a stable base. Hold a light weight (a water bottle works great) in each hand to begin. If you have any shoulder or back concerns, consider performing this exercise without weights to ensure safety.

2. Extend your arms to the side, reaching out at shoulder level. This stance not only prepares your muscles for the exercise but also aids in maintaining balance.

3. Gently lean to your left side, guiding the weight towards the floor in a controlled manner. This action targets the obliques, engaging the side core muscles.

4. Smoothly return to your starting position, keeping your movements measured and your core engaged.

5. Repeat the motion on your right side, ensuring an even and balanced workout.

6. Continue to alternate sides, aiming for 10-15 repetitions on each side. This repetition range is designed to effectively work the muscles without overexertion.

•••Poses for Heart Health and Stamina

Targeted Areas:
Abdominal muscles and obliques.

Benefits:

An excellent exercise for seniors aiming to strengthen their core and improve overall flexibility.

Safety Precautions:

- Move in a controlled manner to avoid strain on the lower back.
- Not recommended for those with acute lower back pain.

Steps:

1. Sit at the edge of a stable chair, leaning back slightly with hands gripping the sides for support. This starting position helps maintain balance and ensures safety throughout the exercise.

2. Gently lift your feet off the ground, engaging your core to stabilize your body.

3. Simulate a cycling motion by alternately bringing one knee towards your chest and extending the other leg forward. This movement should be performed smoothly and at a comfortable pace to avoid any strain. Continue this pedaling action for 30 seconds to 1 minute. Focus on maintaining a steady rhythm, which helps with coordination and keeps the core engaged without overexertion.

SEATED SCISSOR LEGS

Targeted Areas:
Abdominal muscles, hips, and legs.

Benefits:

A fantastic exercise for seniors aiming to strengthen their core, improve leg mobility, and boost coordination.

Safety Precautions:

- Move in a controlled manner to prevent strain.
- Suitable for those looking for a low-impact leg exercise.

Steps:

1. Sit on the edge of your chair, ensuring you're leaning slightly back. This posture helps engage your core throughout the exercise. Use your hands to hold onto the sides of the chair for added support and balance.

2. Carefully lift your feet off the floor, extending your legs in front of you. This initial extension is crucial for preparing your muscles for the scissor movement.

3. Gradually open your legs as wide as comfortable, then cross one leg over the other, alternating legs in a smooth, scissor-like motion. This action not only strengthens the core but also works the leg muscles and hip joints.

4. Continue this alternating leg movement for 30 seconds to 1 minute, depending on your comfort and capability. Focus on maintaining controlled, deliberate motions to maximize the exercise's benefits while minimizing the risk of strain.

Targeted Areas:
Chest, shoulders, and upper back.

Benefits:

An excellent exercise for seniors looking to open up their chest and shoulders, improve their posture, and enhance their breathing.

Safety Precautions:

- Extend your arms and legs to a comfortable degree.
- Ideal for those seeking to improve upper body flexibility.

Steps:

1. Begin by sitting upright in a chair, ensuring your feet are planted flat on the floor for stability.

2. Gently extend your arms and legs outward from your body to form a star shape. This act of extension encourages the opening of the chest and the stretching of the shoulders.

3. Reach through your fingertips and stretch your toes away from the center of your body, intensifying the stretch across your chest and shoulders. This movement not only improves flexibility but also helps to strengthen the muscles involved.

4. Hold this expansive, star-like position for a few deep breaths, focusing on opening your chest with each inhalation and maintaining a strong, extended posture throughout the duration.

5. Gradually relax back to a neutral position, allowing your arms and legs to return to their starting positions.

Seated Knee-to-Chest Lifts with Side Stretch

Targeted Areas:
Abdominal muscles, hips, and thighs.

Benefits:

This exercise is ideal for those seeking to strengthen their lower body in a seated, low-impact manner. It focuses on strengthening the core, improving hip mobility, and building lower body strength.

Safety Precautions:

- Perform knee lifts gently to avoid hip strain.

- Ensure the chair is stable to prevent slipping or tipping.

Steps:

1. Begin by sitting upright in a chair with your feet flat on the floor, creating a stable base for the exercise.

2. Gently lift one knee towards your chest, using your hands for support. If comfortable, gently pull the knee closer to your body to enhance the stretch in the hip and engage the core muscles further.

3. Hold this knee-to-chest position for a few seconds, actively engaging your abdominal muscles to deepen the core workout.

4. For the bonus side stretch, slowly hug the knee out to the side of your body, aiming to keep your back straight and engaging your side muscles for an added stretch. This movement not only aids in hip mobility but also stretches the side abdominal muscles, enhancing flexibility.

5. Carefully return the leg to the starting position, maintaining control and stability.

6. Repeat the knee-to-chest lift and side stretch with the opposite leg, ensuring an even workout on both sides. Alternate legs for 10-15 repetitions per leg to achieve a balanced strengthening and stretching session.

"Gradually Increase Hold Times"

As comfort with poses grows, gradually increase the hold time for each pose. Longer holds can improve strength and flexibility, as well as mental endurance and focus.

SEATED CLAPPING HANDS

Targeted Areas:
Arms, shoulders, and coordination.

Benefits:

An invigorating exercise designed for seniors to improve hand-eye coordination, stimulate blood flow to the arms, and provide an energizing boost.

Safety Precautions:

- Clap at a comfortable pace to avoid straining your wrists.
- Ideal for those looking for a gentle upper body exercise.

Steps:

1. Begin by sitting upright in a chair, ensuring your feet are flat on the ground for stability.

2. Extend your arms in front of you at shoulder height, preparing your upper body for the exercise.

3. Bring your hands together in a clap, then open them wide as if embracing the space around you. This motion encourages blood flow and engages the muscles in your arms and shoulders.

4. Continue this clapping motion in a rhythmic manner for 30 seconds to 1 minute, depending on your comfort level. The goal is to maintain a steady pace that feels energizing without causing strain on your wrists or arms.

Targeted Areas:
Shoulders, arms, and upper back.

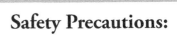

Benefits:

Designed to improve hand-eye coordination, stimulate blood flow to the arms, and provide an energizing boost.

Safety Precautions:

- Swing your arms gently to avoid shoulder strain.
- Ideal for warming up the upper body.

Steps:

1. Sit upright in a chair with your feet flat on the floor, ensuring stability.

2. Allow your arms to hang naturally at your sides. Relax and releasing any tension.

3. Begin by gently swinging your arms forward and upward. As your arms reach shoulder height or slightly higher, keep your movements controlled and fluid.

4. Let your arms swing back and downward, completing the full range of motion.

5. Maintain a natural breathing pattern. Inhale as your arms swing forward and upward, and exhale as they swing back and downward.

6. Continue the arm swings for 30 seconds to 1 minute, depending on your comfort level and fitness. Start with a shorter duration and gradually increase as you build strength and endurance.

INTERMEDIATE 28-DAY CHAIR YOGA CHALLENGE

In the Intermediate challenge, you'll explore a deeper level of chair yoga, ideal for those who have a basic grounding in the practice. These next 28 days are about enhancing your physical capabilities and further alleviating discomfort. As you progress, you'll notice an even greater improvement in your balance, increased flexibility, as well as a reduction in stress, contributing to your overall mental wellness. By the end of the 28 days you will be more independent and confident your daily life.

To start, choose your program: Structured Daily Plan (page 153) or À La Carte Flexible Plan (page 165).

Instructions:

Here are the steps to get started with your chair yoga practice:

1. **Begin each day with a breathing exercise.** This will help to center your mind and prepare your body for the chair yoga session. Found on page 35.

2. **Follow the sequence of poses as outlined for each day.** For Week 1, hold each pose for 30 seconds. Increase this to 40 seconds in Week 2, 45 seconds in Week 3, and 50 seconds in Week 4.

3. **Take a short pause of 15 seconds between each exercise or pose.** Use this time to breathe normally and prepare for the next pose.

4. **Remember to go at your own pace.** It's important to listen to your body and not push beyond comfort. If you experience any discomfort, modify the pose or skip it as needed.

5. **Begin with the goal of practicing these chair yoga workouts daily.** I know that you're busy, but I've found that this consistent approach helps students to establish a routine and maximize the benefits of the program.

   » However, it's important to listen to your body and be mindful of your energy levels and physical comfort.

   » If you find that daily practice is too demanding, or if you experience any discomfort, it's perfectly fine to adjust your schedule.

   » In such cases, aim to complete the workouts 4 to 5 times a week instead.

   » This adjustment ensures that you still maintain regular practice while giving your body adequate time to rest and recover.

I'm here to support you on your journey to a healthier, happier life. If you have any questions, concerns, or would like a few words of encouragement, please don't hesitate to reach out (jcharrisonbooks@gmail.com).

Ending Each Session:

When you're finished with your yoga practice, take a few moments to meditate. This will help you to calm your mind and body and to integrate the benefits of your practice.

» Sit in a comfortable position in your chair. Close your eyes and take a few deep breaths. Focus on your breath, and let go of any thoughts or worries that come to mind.

» After a few minutes, you may want to try a simple meditation technique, such as focusing on a mantra or visualization. Or, you can simply sit quietly and enjoy the feeling of relaxation. For the meditation chapter, see page 239.

» When you're ready, open your eyes and slowly come back to the present moment. Take a few moments to appreciate the sense of relaxation and well-being that you've created.

Breathing Exercise: Three-Part Breath (3 minutes) p. 37

Wrist & Ankle Rotation	Tree Pose	High Lunge	Seated Triangle	Seated Warrior II
30s (p. 43)	30s (p. 127)	30s (p. 123)	30s (p. 134)	30s (p. 132)

DAY 2: HEART HEALTH AND STAMINA

Breathing Exercise: Ocean Breath (3 minutes) p. 38

Toe and Heel Lifts	Twist with Arms	Bicycle	Star Pose	Knee-to-Chest
30s (p. 46)	30s (p. 141)	30s (p. 145)	30s (p. 147)	30s (p. 148)

DAY 3: WEIGHT LOSS FOCUS

Breathing Exercise: Box Breathing (3 minutes) p. 42

Shoulder Stretch	Boxing Punches	Bends w/Weights	Clapping Hands	Squat to Stand
30s (p. 45)	30s (p. 137)	30s (p. 143)	30s (p. 150)	30s (p. 140)

DAY 4: POSTURE IMPROVEMENT

Breathing Exercise: Alternate Nostril Breathing (3 minutes) p. 39

Side Neck Stretch	Mtn Chest Opener	Butterfly	Upward Dog	Forward Fold
30s (p. 45)	30s (p. 111)	30s (p. 114)	30s (p. 115)	30s (p. 112)

DAY 5: MOBILITY

Breathing Exercise: Lion's Breath (3 minutes) p. 40

Toe and Heel Lifts	Side-to-Side Lean	Pigeon Pose	Chair Twist	Eagle Legs
30s (p. 46)	30s (p. 124)	30s (p. 120)	30s (p. 119)	30s (p. 121)

DAY 6: FLEXIBILITY AND BALANCE

Breathing Exercise: Cooling Breath (3 minutes) p. 41

Gentle Backbend	Tree Pose	Seated Warrior II	Seated Dancer	Chair Lotus
30s (p. 46)	30s (p. 127)	30s (p. 132)	30s (p. 122)	30s (p. 131)

Breathing Exercise: Diaphragmatic Breathing (3 minutes) p. 36

Seated Neck Rolls	Bicycle	Supported Chair	Bends w/Weights	Clapping Hands
30s (p. 47)	30s (p. 145)	30s (p. 142)	30s (p. 143)	30s (p. 150)

DAY 8: LOWER BODY FOCUS

Breathing Exercise: Three-Part Breath (3 minutes) p. 37

Wrist & Ankle Rotation	Seated Triangle	Scissor Legs	Squat to Stand	Seated Warrior II
40s (p. 43)	40s (p. 134)	40s (p. 146)	40s (p. 140)	40s (p. 132)

DAY 9: UPPER BODY AND POSTURE

Breathing Exercise: Box Breathing (3 minutes) p. 42

Shoulder Stretch	Forward Fold	Wrist Stretch	Upward Dog	Twist with Arms
40s (p. 45)	40s (p. 112)	40s (p. 116)	40s (p. 115)	40s (p. 141)

Intermediate 28 Day Chair Yoga Challenge - 157

DAY 10: CORE STRENGTH AND FLEXIBILITY

Breathing Exercise: Ocean Breath (3 minutes) p. 38

Shoulder Stretch	Downward Dog	Bicycle	Seated Warrior II	Bends w/Weights
40s (p. 45)	40s (p. 130)	40s (p. 145)	40s (p. 132)	40s (p. 143)

DAY 11: MOBILITY AND STAMINA

Breathing Exercise: Box Breathing (3 minutes) p. 42

Toe and Heel Lifts	Star Pose	Twist with Arms	Arm Swings	Pigeon Pose
40s (p. 46)	40s (p. 147)	40s (p. 141)	40s (p. 151)	40s (p. 120)

DAY 12: BALANCE AND POSTURE

Breathing Exercise: Alternate Nostril Breathing (3 minutes) p. 39

Wrist & Ankle Rotation	Tree Pose	Mtn Chest Opener	High Lunge	Goddess
40s (p. 43)	40s (p. 127)	40s (p. 111)	40s (p. 123)	40s (p. 128)

Breathing Exercise: Lion's Breath (3 minutes) p. 40

Gentle Backbend	Scissor Legs	Knee-to-Chest	Star Pose	Clapping Hands
40s (p. 46)	40s (p. 146)	40s (p. 148)	40s (p. 147)	40s (p. 150)

DAY 14: FLEXIBILITY AND RELAXATION

Breathing Exercise: Cooling Breath (3 minutes) p. 41

Shoulder Stretch	Boxing Punches	Clapping Hands	Squat to Stand	Downward Dog
40s (p. 45)	40s (p. 137)	40s (p. 150)	40s (p. 140)	40s (p. 130)

DAY 15: LOWER BODY AND CORE

Breathing Exercise: Diaphragmatic Breathing (3 minutes) p. 36

Gentle Twists	Butterfly	Warrior I Prayer Hands	Bicycle	Scissor Legs
45s (p. 44)	45s (p. 114)	45s (p. 113)	45s (p. 145)	45s (p. 146)

DAY 16: UPPER BODY AND MOBILITY

Breathing Exercise: Three-Part Breath (3 minutes) p. 37

Side Neck Stretch	Eagle Legs	Seated Dancer	Chair Twist	Upward Dog
45s (p. 45)	45s (p. 121)	45s (p. 122)	45s (p. 119)	45s (p. 115)

DAY 17: POSTURE AND FLEXIBILITY

Breathing Exercise: Box Breathing (3 minutes) p. 42

Shoulder Stretch	Salutation Flow II	Mtn Chest Opener	Goddess	Chair Lotus
45s (p. 45)	1-2 times (p. 138)	45s (p. 111)	45s (p. 128)	45s (p. 131)

DAY 18: BALANCE AND CORE STRENGTH

Breathing Exercise: Ocean Breath (3 minutes) p. 38

Gentle Backbend	Tree Pose	High Lunge	Twist with Arms	Supported Chair
45s (p. 46)	45s (p. 127)	45s (p. 123)	45s (p. 141)	45s (p. 142)

Breathing Exercise: Lion's Breath (3 minutes) p. 40

Gentle Twists	Knee-to-Chest	Scissor Legs	Star Pose	Clapping Hands
45s (p. 44)	45s (p. 148)	45s (p. 146)	45s (p. 147)	45s (p. 150)

DAY 20: MOBILITY AND UPPER BODY

Breathing Exercise: Cooling Breath (3 minutes) p. 41

Seated Neck Rolls	Side-to-Side Lean	Pigeon Pose	Chair Twist	Arm Swings
45s (p. 47)	45s (p. 124)	45s (p. 120)	45s (p. 119)	45s (p. 151)

DAY 21: WEIGHT LOSS AND CARDIO

Breathing Exercise: Diaphragmatic Breathing (3 minutes) p. 36

Wrist & Ankle Rotation	Boxing Punches	Supported Chair	Bicycle	Bends w/Weights
45s (p. 43)	45s (p. 137)	45s (p. 142)	45s (p. 145)	45s (p. 143)

Day 22: Posture and Core Focus

Breathing Exercise: Alternate Nostril Breathing (3 minutes) p. 39

Seated Neck Rolls	Mtn Chest Opener	Butterfly	Forward Fold	Upward Dog
50s (p. 47)	50s (p. 111)	50s (p. 114)	50s (p. 112)	50s (p. 115)

Day 23: Flexibility and Balance

Breathing Exercise: Three-Part Breath (3 minutes) p. 37

Side Neck Stretch	Arm Swings	Seated Warrior II	Goddess	Seated Dancer
50s (p. 45)	50s (p. 151)	50s (p. 132)	50s (p. 128)	50s (p. 122)

Day 24: Heart Health and Mobility

Breathing Exercise: Ocean Breath (3 minutes) p. 38

Gentle Backbend	Twist with Arms	Star Pose	Eagle Legs	Scissor Legs
50s (p. 46)	50s (p. 141)	50s (p. 147)	50s (p. 121)	50s (p. 146)

Breathing Exercise: Box Breathing (3 minutes) p. 42

Gentle Twists	Squat to Stand	Salutation Flow II	Knee-to-Chest	High Lunge
50s (p. 44)	50s (p. 140)	2-3 times (p. 138)	50s (p. 148)	50s (p. 123)

DAY 26: MOBILITY AND RELAXATION

Breathing Exercise: Lion's Breath (3 minutes) p. 40

Wrist & Ankle Rotation	Side-to-Side Lean	Pigeon Pose	Chair Twist	Seated Triangle
50s (p. 43)	50s (p. 124)	50s (p. 120)	50s (p. 119)	50s (p. 134)

DAY 27: UPPER BODY AND CORE STRENGTH

Breathing Exercise: Cooling Breath (3 minutes) p. 41

Shoulder Stretch	Downward Dog	Chair Lotus	Upward Dog	Star Pose
50s (p. 45)	50s (p. 130)	50s (p. 131)	50s (p. 115)	50s (p. 147)

Diaphragmatic Breathing	Warm-up	Review and practice	Closing
	Choose two of your favorite warm-ups to revisit	Choose your favorite poses to revisit	Relaxation and reflection session
3 minutes (p. 36)	50s each.	50s each.	

Week-by-Week Guide

Welcome to the 28-Day Intermediate Flex Plan for Chair Yoga, here is how to get the most from this program over the next 28 days.

Getting Started:

» **Breathing and Warm-Up:** Before you begin, choose 1 breathing and 1 warm-up exercise, from Chapter Three (page 35), to start each day.

» **Choose Your Poses:** Each day, pick 3 or 4 poses that feel comfortable and enjoyable.

» **Flexibility in Your Routine:** Feel free to vary your poses daily. Adjust the duration to suit your energy levels and comfort.

» **Proceed at Your Pace:** Once your poses are selected, you're ready to continue with the program at a pace that feels right for you.

Remember: This journey is all about your wellness and flexibility, tailored to your unique needs and preferences. Let's take this step together, embracing health and joy at every turn!

28-Day Intermediate Flex Plan Chair Yoga Program

Week 1: Dynamic Stretches and Strength Building

» Duration per Pose: 30 seconds.

» Daily Session Length: Start with 10 minutes.

» Focus: Introduce more dynamic stretches and strength-building exercises.

» Breathing Exercises: Begin and end with diaphragmatic breathing.

Week 2: Lower Body and Balance

» Duration per Pose: 40 seconds.

» Daily Session Length: Aim for 12-15 minutes.

» Focus: Greater emphasis on leg strengthening and balance poses.

» Breathing Exercises: Box breathing for relaxation before and after the session.

Week 3: Mobility and Posture

» Duration per Pose: 45 seconds.

» Daily Session Length: Maintain at 15 minutes.

» Focus: Incorporate more standing poses using the chair for support, and add gentle backbends.

» Breathing Exercises: Alternate nostril breathing for focus and balance.

Week 4: Strength, Flexibility and Balance

» Duration per Pose: 50 seconds.

» Daily Session Length: Extend to 18-20 minutes.

» Focus: A comprehensive blend of strength, flexibility, and balance. Introduce more challenging variations.

» Breathing Exercises: Ujjayi breath (ocean breath) to enhance concentration and relaxation.

You are never too old to set another goal or to dream a new dream.

– C.S. Lewis

CHAPTER 6
ADVANCED 28-DAY
CHAIR YOGA CHALLENGE

Chapter Six is where your chair yoga practice intensifies, tailored for those of you who've mastered the basics and are ready for a challenge. This section focuses on advanced poses to further improve your strength, flexibility, and balance. These exercises are designed to support your more exciting daily activities, making them easier and more enjoyable.

This chapter encourages you to push your limits safely and confidently, using your chair as a tool to explore deeper stretches and more complex movements. As you progress, remember the goal is to enhance your overall well-being and maintain your independence, allowing you to enjoy your activities and hobbies with less discomfort and more vitality.

The Advanced 28 Day Challenge can be found on page 222.

POSES FOR BETTER POSTURE

SEATED REVOLVED HEAD TO KNEE POSE

Benefits:

It focuses on stretching the side torso, hamstrings, and shoulders, making it particularly beneficial for seniors looking to maintain or improve their range of motion.

Safety Precautions:

- Stretch gently without straining.
- If you have hip or hamstring issues, moderate the stretch.

Steps:

1. Begin by sitting on a chair, with your legs extended wide apart in front of you. This position allows for a deep stretch without putting strain on your lower back.

2. Gently turn your torso towards your right leg, preparing your body for the side stretch. This rotation starts the engagement of your side torso muscles.

3. Inhale deeply and raise both arms overhead, creating length in your spine and preparing for the stretch. As you exhale, lean towards your right foot, extending your arms as if trying to reach your toes. Keep both arms extended to maximize the stretch along your side body.

4. Hold this position for several deep breaths, focusing on the stretch along your right side. The holding phase allows your muscles to gently elongate and relax, enhancing flexibility.

5. To come out of the pose, inhale and slowly lift your torso, bringing your arms back overhead. Then, gently turn your torso back to center and prepare to repeat the stretch on the opposite side, targeting your left leg.

CHAIR REVERSE WARRIOR

Targeted Areas:
Legs, arms, and side torso.

Benefits:

A gentle yet effective exercise designed for seniors to stretch the side body, strengthen the legs, and enhance flexibility.

Safety Precautions:

• Ensure the chair is stable.

• Be mindful of your balance to avoid straining.

Steps:

1. Begin by standing to the side of the chair, with the chair on your left side for support. Grasp the back of the chair with your left hand to ensure stability.

2. Step your right foot forward into a lunge, bend your right knee so it aligns directly over your right ankle. Keep your left leg straight and strong, ground the heel.

3. Carefully lean your torso back slightly, extending your right arm up and over your head to create a gentle arc with your body. This movement stretches the side torso and engages the legs.

4. Turn your gaze upwards, looking towards your right hand. This not only enhances the stretch but also aids in improving balance and focus.

5. Maintain this pose for a few deep breaths, concentrating on the stretch and strength being cultivated in the pose.

6. To exit the pose, gently straighten your torso and release your right arm down, step back to the starting position. Switch sides, repeat the steps with left foot forward.

Targeted Areas:
Lower back, spine, and shoulders.

Benefits:

Offers a safe and accessible way for seniors to strengthen their back muscles, improve posture, and increase spinal flexibility.

Safety Precautions:

- Move slowly and avoid overstraining your back.
- Not recommended for those with severe back pain.

Steps:

1. Start by sitting at the edge of your chair, ensuring your feet are firmly planted on the floor. This position helps maintain balance and provides a solid foundation.

2. Place your hands on your thighs or beside your hips, depending on what feels most comfortable and provides the best support for the upward movement.

3. As you inhale, gently arch your back, focusing on lifting your chest and shoulders upwards and backwards. This motion mimics the Locust Pose's back extension, activating the muscles in the lower back and spine.

4. For those who can and wish to deepen the stretch, extend your arms behind you, reaching away from your back. This optional step increases the intensity of the stretch, further engaging the back muscles and shoulders.

5. Hold this position for several deep breaths, concentrating on the stretching and strengthening sensations throughout your back.

6. To release, exhale, slowly return, allow your back to relax before repeating if desired.

SEATED FISH POSE

Targeted Areas:
Spine, chest, shoulders, throat, and thyroid.

Benefits:

This variation enhances spinal flexibility, opens the chest and shoulders, and stimulates the throat and thyroid gland.

Safety Precautions:

- Ensure your chair is stable and will not slide.

- Be mindful to lift the chest and open the shoulders without straining the neck.

- If you experience any discomfort in your lower back, adjust your hand placement or reduce the backbend.

SEATED FISH POSE

Steps:

1. Begin in a seated mountain pose, sitting upright with your feet pressed firmly into the floor and your spine lengthened.

2. Place your hands on your hips, lower back, or with fingertips on the seat of the chair behind you, fingers pointing forward, depending on what feels most comfortable and supportive.

3. Draw your shoulder blades toward each other, lifting your sternum to open the chest.

4. You may keep your feet in the sitting mountain position or extend your legs, pressing into the bottom of your feet and engaging your thighs for added stability and stretch.

5. Lift your chin slightly, directing your gaze towards the seam where the roof meets the wall, creating a gentle extension in the neck.

6. If comfortable, lean back slightly and press into your palms or the seat of the chair to deepen the chest expansion. Ensure this movement is gradual and controlled to avoid straining the back.

7. Optionally, you can extend your lower jaw forward and smile gently. This action activates the throat and front of the neck, enhancing the stretch without compressing the back of the neck.

8. Breathe deeply into the front of your torso, allowing the breath to facilitate a deeper opening in the chest and shoulders.

9. To come out of the pose, slowly lift your torso back to an upright seated position. Sit quietly for a breath or two, allowing your body to integrate the effects of the pose.

CHAIR DOWNWARD DOG POSE

Targeted Areas:
Hamstrings, shoulders, and back.

Benefits:

It stretches the back, strengthens the arms and legs, and offers a calming effect on the mind.

Safety Precautions:

- Ensure the chair is stable.
- Avoid if you have severe wrist or shoulder pain.

Steps:

1. Begin by standing in front of a chair, feet hip-width apart, ensuring the chair is stable and secure. This precaution is crucial for maintaining safety throughout the pose.

2. Lean forward and place your hands on the seat of the chair. Carefully step back until your body forms an inverted 'V' shape. This positioning uses the chair to support your upper body, making the pose accessible and safe.

3. Aim to keep your spine and legs straight, creating a long line from your hands through your spine and down to your hips. This alignment helps in stretching the back and legs effectively.

4. Gently press your chest towards your thighs, deepening the stretch along your back and hamstrings. This movement also aids in strengthening your arms by bearing some of your body's weight.

5. Hold this position for several deep breaths, focusing on the stretch and the calming rhythm of your breathing. The duration of the hold helps in maximizing the stretch and the calming benefits of the pose.

6. To release, slowly walk your feet forward, coming back to a standing position and then relax. This gradual movement helps in avoiding any sudden strain on the muscles.

UPWARD PLANK

Benefits:

The Upward Plank using a chair offers a modified approach to strengthen the arms, shoulders, back, and improve core stability. It's tailored for seniors, focusing on enhancing upper body strength and core stability without the need for floor exercises.

Safety Precautions:

- Ensure the chair is stable and won't slip.
- Avoid if you have wrist or shoulder injuries.

Steps:

1. Start by sitting on the edge of a stable chair, placing your hands firmly beside your hips for support. This initial position is crucial for ensuring safety and stability throughout the exercise.

2. Carefully slide your buttocks off the chair, using your hands to support your weight. This movement requires engaging your arm and shoulder muscles, providing a solid foundation for the pose.

3. Extend your legs straight in front of you, resting your heels on the ground. This leg position helps in creating a stable base and adds to the intensity of the core and leg engagement.

4. Press down through your hands and lift your hips towards the ceiling, aiming to form a straight line from your head to your heels. This action engages the core, back, and shoulders, strengthening these key areas.

5. Hold this position for several breaths, focusing on maintaining a solid and stable form. The holding phase is essential for building strength and stability in the targeted areas.

6. To finish, gently lower your hips back to the chair, moving slowly and with control to avoid any strain.

POSES FOR MOBILITY

Targeted Areas:
Legs, hips, and chest.

Benefits:

The Chair Warrior I Variation is a tailored exercise for seniors, focusing on strengthening the legs, enhancing balance, and opening the hips and chest.

Safety Precautions:

- Ensure the chair is stable and doesn't slide.
- Avoid overstraining the back leg.

Steps:

1. Begin by standing behind a chair, using the back of the chair for support. This ensures stability and safety throughout the exercise.

2. Step your right foot forward, bending the knee to create a lunge position. Ensure your left leg remains straight with the heel firmly planted on the ground, providing a stretch through the back leg.

3. As you find your balance, lift your arms overhead. You can choose to join your palms for added stretch through the upper body or keep them shoulder-width apart if that's more comfortable.

4. Focus your gaze straight ahead or slightly upwards, aligning your posture and deepening the stretch across your chest and hips. Hold this position for a few deep breaths, allowing your body to settle into the pose.

5. Gently release the pose, returning to your starting position, and then switch legs, repeating the steps with your left leg forward.

SEATED WIDE LEG FORWARD POSE

Targeted Areas:
Inner thighs, hamstrings, and lower back.

Benefits:

This pose is designed for seniors, focusing on stretching the inner thighs and hamstrings, calming the mind, and improving flexibility.

Safety Precautions:

- Move into the forward bend slowly to avoid straining the back.

- If you have hip or hamstring issues, moderate the stretch.

Steps:

1. Begin by sitting on the edge of your chair, providing the freedom to open your legs wide without restriction. This is essential for achieving the maximum benefit.

2. Take a deep breath in to prepare, focusing on elongating your spine. As you exhale, gently hinge forward from your hips, leading with your chest. This technique ensures a safe and effective stretch that targets the intended areas without strain.

3. Lower your torso towards the floor as far as it feels comfortable for you, allowing your hands to rest either on the floor or on your legs. This variation allows for personalization of the stretch based on your current flexibility and comfort level.

4. Maintain this forward bend for several deep breaths, embracing the stretch and the calming effect it has on your mind. The duration of the hold is a crucial aspect, providing ample time for the muscles to relax and lengthen.

5. To conclude the pose, slowly rise back up to a seated position, taking care to move gently to prevent any sudden strain on the back or legs.

Targeted Areas:
Legs, core, and balance.

CHAIR WARRIOR III VARIATION

Benefits:

Designed to enhance balance, strengthen the legs and core, and improve concentration for seniors.

Safety Precautions:

- Use the chair for support to maintain balance.
- Avoid if you have severe balance issues.

Steps:

1. Begin by standing behind a chair, placing your hands securely on the backrest. This provides the necessary support to perform the pose safely, especially for those concerned with balance.

2. Carefully lift your right leg straight behind you. At the same time, lean your torso forward until your body forms a 'T' shape. This action engages the muscles in your standing leg and core, challenging your balance and strengthening these areas.

3. Extend your arms forward, keeping them parallel to the floor. This arm position helps with balance and aligns your body correctly in the pose.

4. Hold this position for several deep breaths, focusing on maintaining stability and alignment. The act of balancing and focusing during this pose enhances concentration and mental clarity.

5. Gently return to your starting position and repeat the exercise with your left leg lifted. This ensures that both sides of the body are worked evenly, maintaining symmetry in muscle strength and flexibility.

CHAIR REVOLVED TRIANGLE POSE

Targeted Areas:
Spine, legs, and core.

Benefits:

This pose enhances spinal flexibility, stimulates abdominal organs, and improves balance and concentration.

Safety Precautions:

- Move into the twist slowly to avoid strain.
- Use the chair for support to maintain balance.

Steps:

1. Begin by standing in front of a chair, feet hip-width apart, facing towards the chair.

2. Step your left foot back about a leg's length, keeping your right foot facing forward. The back foot should be at a 45-degree angle, grounding through the edge of the foot.

3. Inhale and extend your torso over the right leg, placing your hands on the seat of the chair for support. This initial forward bend helps to lengthen the spine and prepare for the twist.

4. As you exhale, initiate the twist to your right, extending your right arm towards the ceiling if balance allows. Your left hand can remain on the chair for support, or for a deeper twist, place it on the outside of your right foot on the chair.

5. Turn your head to gaze up towards your right hand, ensuring your spine is elongated and your twist originates from your mid-torso.

6. Hold the pose for several breaths, focusing on deepening the twist with each exhale while maintaining balance and stability.

7. To come out of the pose, lower your right arm, unwind your torso, and gently stand back up to the starting position.

8. Repeat on the opposite side to maintain balance in the body.

SEATED CRESCENT LUNGE POSE

Targeted Areas:

Hips, thighs, and core.

Benefits:

This pose helps to stretch the hip flexors, enhance lower body strength, and improve balance and stability.

Safety Precautions:

• Ensure the chair is stable.

• Avoid if you have severe knee or hip pain.

"Engage in Active Sitting"

Instead of passively resting on the chair, engage the muscles slightly even when seated. This "active sitting" helps build core strength and keeps the body engaged and ready for movement.

Steps:

1. Begin by sitting at the edge of your chair, turning your legs and body to the left side, ensuring it's stable.

2. Inhale deeply and step your right foot back into a high lunge, positioning the back heel straight up to the sky and bend your front knee to a 90-degree angle, ensuring it is directly above your ankle. This posture starts the engagement and strengthening of your legs.

3. Your back leg should be straight, with the heel lifted off the ground, mimicking the stance of a traditional Crescent Lunge. This engages the thigh muscles of your back leg for stability and a deeper stretch in the hip flexor.

4. Inhale and raise your arms above your head if balance allows, or keep your hands on the chair for support. Engage your core to keep your torso upright and stable.

5. Gently arch your back and open your chest towards the ceiling, creating a slight backbend to enhance the stretch in your chest and front body.

6. Hold the pose for several breaths, focusing on a deep stretch through the hip flexor of the back leg and maintaining balance and stability.

7. To exit the pose, carefully lower your arms (if raised) and step your back foot forward to return to your sitting position.

8. Repeat the pose with the opposite leg forward to ensure a balanced workout.

CHAIR SUPPORTED SUN SALUTATION

Targeted Areas:
Core, legs, arms, spine, shoulders, and hips.

Benefits:

A comprehensive, full-body stretch and strengthening sequence that enhances flexibility, improves circulation, and builds strength.

Safety Precautions:

• Keep your movements smooth and controlled to avoid any strain, particularly when transitioning.

• Adjust the depth of the poses to your comfort level, especially in forward folds and lunges, to prevent overstretching.

Steps:

1. Stand in front of your chair, facing the seat, with arms by your side and feet hip-distance apart. This is your starting position.

2. Inhale and reach your arms up towards the sky, elongating your spine and stretching your entire body.

3. As you exhale, fold forward, bending your knees slightly. Place your hands on the chair seat, letting your head drop to relax your neck and shoulders.

4. Inhale and step your right foot back into a modified Warrior I pose. Keep your left knee bent directly above your left ankle, hips facing forward. Place your hands on the chair for support, lengthening through the spine.

5. Exhale and step your left foot back to join your right, coming into a Downward Dog position with your hands still on the chair. Allow your head to drop between your arms, pulling your hips back.

6. Engage your core and shift your upper body forward into a Plank position, shoulders stacked over your wrists, keeping your body in a straight line supported by the chair.

7. Inhale, and as you exhale, return to your Downward Dog position, extending your arms and pulling your hips back.

8. Step your right foot forward under your chair, returning to a modified Warrior I pose on the opposite side. Take a few breaths in this position.

9. As you exhale, step your left foot forward to meet your right, returning to a forward fold with your hands on the chair, head dropped, and knees bent.

10. Inhale, bend your knees slightly, and with a strong push through your legs, bring yourself back up, sweeping your arms up towards the sky.

11. Exhale and bring your hands to your heart, taking a moment to breathe and prepare to repeat the sequence, this time stepping your left foot back first.

POSES FOR FLEXIBILITY AND BALANCE

Targeted Areas:
Thighs, chest, and balance.

Benefits:

Chair Dancer Pose is a graceful exercise that enhances balance, and focuses on improving mobility and stability.

Safety Precautions:

- Use the chair for stability.
- Avoid if you have knee or balance issues.

Steps:

1. Start by standing beside a chair, using the backrest for support. This will help maintain balance throughout the pose.

2. Bend your right knee and reach back to hold your right foot or ankle with your right hand. This action begins the stretch and prepares your body for the balance aspect.

3. Gently press your foot into your hand, lifting your leg behind you as far as comfortably possible. This movement stretches the thigh and chest while strengthening the standing leg.

4. Keep your other hand on the chair for support, ensuring stability as you focus on maintaining the pose for several breaths. This aids in developing balance and concentration.

5. After holding the pose, gently release your leg and switch sides, repeating the steps with your left leg.

CHAIR HALF MOON BALANCE

Targeted Areas:
Legs, hips, and side torso.

Benefits:

This pose is excellent for improving balance and coordination, strengthening the muscles of the standing leg, and providing a deep stretch along the side of the body.

Safety Precautions:

• Use the chair for support to maintain balance.

• Avoid if you have balance or lower body mobility issues.

CHAIR HALF MOON BALANCE

Steps:

1. Begin by standing with your left side next to the chair, placing your left hand on the backrest for support. This ensures stability as you enter the pose.

2. Carefully shift your weight onto your left leg, grounding through the foot for balance. This activates the muscles in the standing leg, preparing them for the pose.

3. Gradually lift your right leg to the side, keeping it straight, while simultaneously tilting your torso to the left. Aim to create a straight line from your left foot through your torso and out through your right fingertips, which are reaching towards the sky.

4. As you balance, extend your right arm upward, directly in line with your left leg. This action not only enhances the stretch along the right side of your body but also encourages a strong sense of balance and alignment.

5. Maintain this position for a few deep, steady breaths, focusing on the stretch and strength being cultivated in the pose.

6. To exit, gently lower your right leg back to the ground and return to a standing position before switching sides to ensure a balanced practice.

SEATED HUMBLE WARRIOR POSE VARIATION

Targeted Areas:
Hip flexors, thighs, core, spine, and posture.

Benefits:

Enhancing flexibility, stability, and strength in a seated position, while also improving posture and spinal alignment.

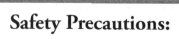

Safety Precautions:

- Ensure the chair is stable and secure to prevent shifting or tipping.
- Keep the front knee aligned over the ankle to avoid straining the knee joint.
- Engage your core throughout the pose to support your spine and maintain balance.
- Adjust the depth of the pose to your comfort level to prevent overstretching.

Steps:

1. Start by sitting upright towards the front edge of a stable chair, feet flat on the ground, turning your legs and body to the left side.

2. Slide your right leg back, planting your foot at a 45 to 60-degree angle to the front and your leg extended straight behind you, simulating the Warrior I leg stance. Bend your left knee, positioning it directly over your left ankle.

3. Rest both hands gently on your left (front) thigh. This action helps to stabilize your upper body and maintain a focused engagement with the pose.

4. Engage your core and lengthen your spine, drawing your shoulders down and away from your ears to maintain an open, upright posture.

5. Gently press your hands into your thigh, encouraging a slight forward lean in the torso while keeping your back straight. This position intensifies the stretch in the hip flexor of the back leg and engages the muscles in the front thigh.

6. Hold this position for several deep breaths, focusing on the sensation of stretching and strengthening in the legs and hips. Maintain a grounded feeling through both feet, especially the front foot, to enhance stability.

7. To release the pose, gently lift your torso, remove your hands from your thigh, and return your back leg to the starting position.

8. Repeat on the opposite side, extending the left leg back and bending the right knee, to ensure an even stretch and strengthening across both sides of the body.

Seated Extended Side Angle Pose

Targeted Areas:
Spine, side torso, shoulders, neck, and hips.

Benefits:

Helps improve flexibility in the spine and hips, enhances circulation, and can aid in alleviating stiffness.

Safety Precautions:

• Ensure the chair is stable and secure to prevent it from moving.

• Move into and out of the pose gently to avoid any sudden movements that could lead to discomfort or injury.

• Listen to your body and only stretch as far as comfortably possible without straining.

Steps:

1. Begin by sitting upright in a chair, feet flat on the floor, spaced hip-width apart. Ensure your back is straight, and you're positioned towards the front of the chair for greater freedom of movement.

2. Extend your right leg out to the side, keeping your left foot planted firmly on the ground opening your hips as far as it feels comfortable. If possible, rotate your right foot so that it points slightly outward, aligning with the direction of your stretch.

3. Inhale and raise your right arm overhead, extending it alongside your ear. Keep your left hand on your left thigh.

4. As you exhale, gently lean your torso to the left, gently resting your forearm over the left thigh. Extend your right arm further to enhance the stretch along the right side of your body. Keep your chest open and your gaze directed forward or slightly upwards, maintaining a long, straight line from your right fingertips down to your right hip.

5. Maintain this position for several deep breaths, focusing on the stretch along the right side of your torso. With each exhale, try to deepen the stretch slightly, without pushing beyond your comfort level.

6. To release, inhale and gently come back to an upright seated position, lowering your right arm. Bring your right leg back to the starting position.

7. Repeat on the Opposite Side: Extend your left leg out, and repeat the stretch on the other side to ensure balance in the stretch and flexibility.

STANDING CHAIR EAGLE POSE

Targeted Areas:
Legs, hips, and balance.

Benefits:

Improving balance, strengthening the legs, and improving focus.

Safety Precautions:

- Use the chair for support to maintain balance.
- Avoid if you have knee or balance issues.

STANDING CHAIR EAGLE POSE

Steps:

1. Begin by standing in front of a chair, keeping your feet together to ensure a stable starting position. The chair will serve as your support throughout the pose.

2. Slightly bend your knees and cross your right thigh over your left thigh. This action starts to engage your legs and hips, preparing them for the balance challenge.

3. Attempt to hook your right foot behind your left calf, if possible. This adds to the pose's complexity, increasing the balance and strength required. However, it's essential to only go as far as is comfortable for you.

4. Cross your arms in front of your chest, placing your left arm over your right. Then, press your palms together, or as close as possible, to enhance the stretch and balance component of the pose.

5. Hold this position for several breaths, focusing on maintaining your balance and the alignment of your pose. Use the chair for support as needed to ensure safety.

6. Gently unwind from the pose and switch sides, repeating the steps with the opposite leg and arm to maintain symmetry in your exercise routine.

CHAIR SUPPORTED WARRIOR II

Benefits:

Chair Supported Warrior II is an exercise designed for seniors to fortify the legs and arms, enhance concentration, and boost stamina.

Safety Precautions:

- Ensure proper alignment to avoid strain.
- Avoid if you have hip or knee injuries.

CHAIR SUPPORTED WARRIOR II

Steps:

1. Begin by standing behind your chair, using the back for support. This position ensures stability and safety throughout the exercise.

2. Step your feet wide apart, establishing a solid base. Turn your right foot outwards and your left foot to face forward, setting up the foundational stance for Warrior II.

3. Bend your left knee, aiming to align it directly over your ankle. This alignment is crucial for protecting the knee joint and ensuring the exercise's effectiveness.

4. Straighten your right leg, pressing the outer edge of your right foot into the floor for stability. This action engages the leg muscles and helps maintain balance.

5. Extend your right arm back to shoulder height, parallel to the floor, while keeping your left hand on the chair. Turn your head to gaze over your left arm, focusing on a point that helps maintain balance and concentration.

6. Hold this position for several deep breaths, feeling the strength and stretch in your legs and arms. This hold is vital for building stamina and improving concentration.

7. Carefully release the pose and switch sides, repeating the steps with your right leg bent and your left arm extended to ensure a balanced workout.

POSES FOR WEIGHT LOSS

SEATED MOUNTAIN CLIMBERS

Benefits:

A dynamic way to boost the heart rate, strengthen the core, and enhance lower body mobility.

Safety Precautions:

- Move at a pace that is challenging but maintains your balance.
- Ideal for those seeking a cardio workout from a seated position.

Steps:

1. Begin by sitting at the edge of your chair to allow for greater freedom of movement. Ensure your posture is upright, with your hands resting on the sides of the chair.

2. Engage your core muscles as you lift one knee towards your chest, then quickly switch to lift the other knee, creating a motion similar to running. This movement not only strengthens the core but also mobilizes the hip and knee joints.

3. Continue alternating your knees in a brisk but controlled pace. The rapid movement helps to increase your heart rate, providing a cardiovascular workout.

4. Aim to maintain this activity for 30 seconds to 1 minute, depending on your fitness level and comfort. The key is to find a pace that is challenging yet allows you to maintain balance and control throughout the exercise.

CHAIR PLANK

Targeted Areas:
Obliques, shoulders, and core.

Benefits:

The Chair Plank is a modified exercise designed to strengthen the core, to improve balance and stability.

Safety Precautions:

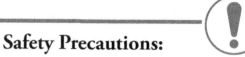

- Perform near a wall or stable surface for additional support if needed.
- Avoid if you have shoulder or wrist pain.

CHAIR PLANK

Steps:

1. Start by placing a stable chair against a wall if needed to ensure it won't move during the exercise.

2. Stand facing the chair, keeping your back straight bend forward from the hips, and place both hands on the seat slightly wider than shoulder-width apart. Ensure your wrists are directly under your shoulders.

3. Step back one foot at a time, extending your legs fully behind you, coming onto the balls of your feet. Your body should form a straight line from your head to your heels, similar to the alignment in a traditional plank pose but elevated.

4. Tighten your abdominal muscles and draw your navel towards your spine to keep your core engaged. This supports your lower back and enhances the strength-building aspect of the plank.

5. Hold the plank position, focusing on maintaining a strong, stable posture. Your gaze should be down and slightly forward to keep your neck in a neutral position.

6. Start with holding the pose for 10-30 seconds, gradually increasing the time as your strength improves.

CHAIR BOAT POSE

Targeted Areas:
Abdominal muscles, hip flexors, balance and focus.

Benefits:

Designed to strengthen the core muscles, improve digestion, and enhance balance and focus.

Safety Precautions:

• Ensure the chair is stable and securely placed on a non-slip surface to prevent any movement.

• Keep your spine straight and long throughout the pose to avoid rounding the back, which can put unnecessary pressure on the lower back.

• Engage your core muscles actively to support your spine and maintain balance.

CHAIR BOAT POSE

Steps:

1. Start by sitting halfway on a stable chair, feet flat on the floor, and hands resting lightly on the sides of the chair or the seat for support.

2. Engage your core muscles by drawing your navel towards your spine, preparing your body for the lift.

3. Lean slightly back in the chair, keeping your back straight and chest lifted to avoid collapsing the spine.

4. Lift your feet off the floor, bringing your shins parallel to the floor, or as high as comfortable, to initiate the Boat Pose.

5. If possible, release your hands from the chair and extend them forward, parallel to the ground, to increase the engagement of the core muscles. Ensure your shoulders are relaxed and away from your ears.

6. Hold the pose for several breaths, focusing on maintaining balance and stability while keeping the core engaged. The intensity of the pose can be increased by holding it longer or by straightening the legs to form a V shape.

7. To exit the pose, gently lower your feet back to the floor and relax your arms, sitting upright to release the pose.

8. Pause for a moment to observe the effects of the pose before continuing with your practice or moving on with your day.

SEATED RUSSIAN TWISTS

Targeted Areas:
Core, especially obliques, and spine.

Benefits:

This exercise targets the core muscles and spine, promoting better posture and flexibility.

Safety Precautions:

- Twist from your torso, not your neck.
- Avoid if you have lower back pain.

Steps:

1. Begin by sitting on the edge of a chair, ensuring you're in a stable position to prevent any strain on your lower back. Lean slightly back, but maintain a straight spine to engage your core effectively.

2. For an added challenge, and only if it feels comfortable, lift your feet slightly off the floor. This increases the engagement of your core muscles throughout the exercise.

3. Place your hands together in front of you for balance. Twist your torso to the right, aiming to touch the chair with your hands, or as close as you comfortably can, to ensure a full twist in your obliques.

4. Then, twist your torso to the left, repeating the motion and ensuring an equal workout on both sides of your core. The movement should come from your waist, avoiding twisting from your neck to prevent strain.

5. Continue alternating sides, performing this twisting motion for 30s to 1 min. Focus on controlled, deliberate movements to maximize benefits to your core and spine.

Targeted Areas:

Arms, chest, and shoulders.

CHAIR PUSH-UPS

Benefits:

Chair Push-Ups are a modified upper body exercise designed for seniors to strengthen the arms, chest, and shoulders.

Safety Precautions:

- Ensure the chair is stable and won't slip.
- Keep your core engaged to protect your lower back.

Steps:

1. Begin by standing in front of a stable chair, ensuring it is securely placed against a wall or on a non-slip surface to prevent movement during the exercise.

2. Place your hands on the seat of the chair, positioning them slightly wider than shoulder-width apart. This hand placement allows for a stable base and targets the upper body muscles effectively.

3. Step your feet back until your body is in a plank position, with your weight evenly distributed between your hands and toes. Keep your body in a straight line from head to heels, engaging your core to support your lower back.

4. Bend your elbows to lower your chest towards the seat of the chair, keeping your elbows close to your body. This motion engages the chest, arms, and shoulders.

5. Push through your hands to lift your body back up to the starting plank position, completing one repetition.

6. Aim for 10-15 repetitions, focusing on maintaining proper form and controlled movements throughout the set.

CHAIR SQUAT JUMPS

Targeted Areas:
Legs, glutes, and cardiovascular system.

Benefits:

Designed to safely build lower body strength, enhance cardiovascular health, and increase leg power for seniors.

Safety Precautions:

• Move softly to protect your knees and ankles.

• Not recommended for those with severe knee or hip issues.

CHAIR SQUAT JUMPS

Steps:

1. Begin by sitting halfway on a stable chair with your feet hip-width apart and flat on the floor. Ensure the chair is securely positioned to prevent any movement during the exercise.

2. Lean slightly forward, engaging your core, and press through your heels to stand up from the chair. As you reach a standing position, extend your arms in front of you for balance.

3. Instead of performing an explosive jump, raise onto the balls of your feet, lifting your heels off the ground. This motion mimics the jump's upward phase, activating the calf muscles and glutes with minimal impact on the joints.

4. Reverse the motion by lowering your heels back to the floor and then slowly bending your knees to return to a seated position on the chair. This controlled descent is crucial for building strength in the thighs and glutes.

5. To add a slight cardiovascular challenge without the impact of a traditional jump, quickly stand again and repeat the heel raise. This rapid succession of movements will help increase your heart rate.

6. Perform 10-15 repetitions of this modified squat to heel raise, focusing on smooth transitions between sitting and standing to maintain balance and engage the targeted muscle groups effectively.

POSES FOR HEART HEALTH AND STAMINA

Targeted Areas:
Chest, back, and spine.

Benefits:

This pose increases strength in your back muscles to reduce back pain and increase spinal flexibility. It's particularly beneficial for improving posture and alleviating the stiffness that comes as we age.

Safety Precautions:

• Use the chair for support and avoid over-arching your back.

• Not recommended for those with severe back pain.

Steps:

1. Begin by positioning yourself behind the chair, ensuring it is stable. Grasp the backrest with both hands for support.

2. Inhale deeply, and as you exhale, gently arch your back. Engage in pushing your hips slightly forward while simultaneously lifting your chest towards the ceiling. This movement encourages an extension of the spine and opens the front of the body.

3. Maintain this arched position for a few deep breaths. Focus on the sensation of expansion across your chest and the gentle strengthening of your back muscles. Ensure to keep the movement within a comfortable range to avoid any strain.

4. To conclude, inhale and gently return to a neutral standing position. Take a moment to observe any shifts in your body.

CHAIR SUPPORTED WARRIOR FLOW

Targeted Areas:
Legs, arms, and spine.

Benefits:

This brings numerous advantages, including improved leg strength, greater flexibility, and enhanced mobility, designed to enrich your daily activities by making movements smoother and more effortless.

Safety Precautions:

- Move smoothly between poses to avoid strain.
- Use the chair for support throughout the flow.

Steps:

1. Begin by sitting at the edge of your chair, turning your legs and body to the left side, ensuring it's stable.

2. Inhale deeply and step your right foot back into a high lunge, positioning the back straight up to the sky and bending the front knee to align over the front ankle. This posture starts the engagement and strengthening of your legs.

3. Smoothly transition into Warrior II by rotating your back foot flat and opening your hips and chest sideways. Extend your arms parallel to the floor, shoulder height, gazing over your front hand. This pose enhances leg strength and opens the hips and chest.

4. For the Reverse Warrior, keep the front knee bent, lift your front arm towards the ceiling, and let your back hand gently rest on the back leg. This action stretches the side of the body, improving flexibility in the spine and sides.

5. After holding the pose for a few breaths, smoothly transition to the other side, repeating the sequence. This balance ensures even strength and flexibility development on both sides of the body.

6. Continue alternating sides for several cycles, moving with your breath. This repetition helps to deepen the poses with each cycle, promoting flexibility and strength.

SEATED HIGH-LEG MARCHES

Targeted Areas:
Legs, hips, and cardiovascular system.

Benefits:

This is an excellent exercise for seniors, designed to improve leg strength and mobility, enhance coordination, and boost cardiovascular health.

Safety Precautions:

- Move in a controlled manner to avoid losing balance.
- Suitable for those seeking a low-impact cardio exercise.

Steps:

1. Begin by sitting upright on a chair, ensuring your feet are flat on the ground. This starting position promotes good posture and stability throughout the exercise.

2. Engage your core muscles to provide additional support for your upper body. Then, lift one knee as high as comfortably possible, mimicking a marching motion. The higher you lift your knee, the more you engage the muscles in your leg and hip.

3. Lower the lifted knee back to the starting position and then lift the other knee, continuing the marching motion. This alternating action helps to evenly work both legs while also promoting coordination and balance.

4. Continue this rhythmic marching motion for 30 seconds to 1 minute, depending on your comfort and fitness level. Focus on maintaining a controlled pace to maximize the cardiovascular benefits without risking balance.

5. As you perform the exercise, breathe evenly and maintain an upright posture to ensure effective engagement of your core and leg muscles.

Targeted Areas:

Thighs, glutes, and lower back.

Benefits:

An effective exercise for seniors designed to improve posture, as well as enhance lower body strength and stability.

Safety Precautions:

- Keep your back straight and avoid leaning too far forward.
- Avoid if you have knee problems.

Steps:

1. Begin by standing in front of a stable chair, ensuring it is securely positioned to avoid any movement. Your feet should be hip-width apart to provide a solid base for the exercise.

2. Slowly bend your knees and lower your hips towards the chair, as if you are about to sit down. Stop the movement just above the seat, creating a hovering position that challenges your thigh and glute muscles.

3. Extend your arms forward, keeping them parallel to the floor. This arm position helps maintain balance and alignment, while also engaging the core and upper body.

4. Hold this position for several deep breaths, focusing on maintaining a straight back and avoiding leaning too far forward to protect your knees and lower back.

5. After holding the pose, press through your heels to stand back up, returning to the starting position.

CHAIR SIDE PLANK

Benefits:

This pose strengthens the arms, shoulders, and core muscles, making it an effective exercise for enhancing core stability, targeting the obliques, and strengthening the shoulders.

Safety Precautions:

• Keep your supporting arm strong and directly under your shoulder to avoid strain.

• Engage your core muscles throughout the exercise to maintain form and protect your lower back.

• If you feel any discomfort or instability, return to the starting position and adjust as necessary.

OPTIONAL

Steps:

1. Position yourself in front of the chair, keeping your back straight bend forward from the hips, and place both hands on the seat wider than shoulder-width apart. Step your feet back to extend your legs behind you, engaging your core to form a straight line from head to heels.

2. Move your left hand to the center of the chair and walk your feet together. Slowly shift your weight onto your left hand while keeping your feet together and rotating your body and opening to the right side. Stack your feet for more challenge, or keep them slightly apart for better balance. Ensure your left shoulder is directly over your left hand for stability.

3. As you balance on your left hand, you can choose to keep your right hand on your hips or lift it towards the ceiling, opening your chest and hips to the side. Your body should form a straight line from head to feet, mirroring the alignment of a traditional side plank.

4. Engage your obliques and keep your hips lifted, maintaining the side plank position. Hold this pose for 10-30 seconds, focusing on stability and core engagement.

5. Carefully rotate your torso back to the chair plank position, placing your right hand back on the chair seat. Ensure control and stability as you transition.

6. Repeat on the Opposite Side. Shift your weight to your right hand and repeat the side plank on the other side to ensure balanced strength development across your core and shoulders.

SEATED OBLIQUE TWISTS WITH A LIGHT WEIGHT

Targeted Areas:
Obliques, core, and spine.

Benefits:

This exercise specifically targets the obliques, core, and spine, contributing to better posture and reducing the risk of lower back pain.

Safety Precautions:

• Use a light weight to avoid strain.

• Twist gently, especially if you have lower back issues.

SEATED OBLIQUE TWISTS WITH A LIGHT WEIGHT

Steps:

1. Begin by sitting upright on a chair with your feet planted firmly on the ground. This stable seated position ensures safety and effectiveness throughout the exercise.

2. Hold a light weight with both hands. This could be a small dumbbell, a water bottle, or any household item that provides a slight resistance without causing strain.

3. Extend your arms in front of you, keeping them at chest height. Ensure your grip on the weight is secure, and your shoulders are relaxed.

4. Gently twist your torso to the left, moving the weight towards the left side. Keep your movements controlled and focused, engaging the muscles on the side of your abdomen.

5. Slowly twist your torso to the right, transferring the weight to the right side. This action continues the engagement of your core muscles, particularly the obliques.

6. Continue alternating twists from left to right for 30 seconds to 1 minute. Focus on maintaining a smooth, controlled motion to maximize the benefits to your obliques and spine.

Advanced 28-Day Chair Yoga Challenge

In the Advanced section you'll explore dynamic poses that significantly boost your strength, balance, and flexibility. This 28-day journey is not just about physical achievements; it's a profound step towards mastering pain management and enhancing mental wellness. Get ready to feel a remarkable sense of accomplishment and empowerment, as you deepen your bonds within the yoga community and stride confidently towards greater independence in your daily life. This is your moment to shine!

To start, choose your program: Structured Daily Plan (page 223) or À La Carte Flexible Plan (page 235).

Instructions:

Here are the steps to get started with your chair yoga practice:

1. **Begin each day with a breathing exercise.** This will help to center your mind and prepare your body for the chair yoga session. Found on page 35.

2. **Follow the sequence of poses as outlined for each day.** For Week 1, hold each pose for 30 seconds. Increase this to 40 seconds in Week 2, 45 seconds in Week 3, and 50 seconds in Week 4.

3. **Take a short pause of 15 seconds between each exercise or pose.** Use this time to breathe normally and prepare for the next pose.

4. **Remember to go at your own pace.** It's important to listen to your body and not push beyond comfort. If you experience any discomfort, modify the pose or skip it as needed.

5. **Begin with the goal of practicing these chair yoga workouts daily.** I know that you're busy, but I've found that this consistent approach helps students to establish a routine and maximize the benefits of the program.

   » However, it's important to listen to your body and be mindful of your energy levels and physical comfort.

   » If you find that daily practice is too demanding, or if you experience any discomfort, it's perfectly fine to adjust your schedule.

   » In such cases, aim to complete the workouts 4 to 5 times a week instead.

   » This adjustment ensures that you still maintain regular practice while giving your body adequate time to rest and recover.

I'm here to support you on your journey to a healthier, happier life. If you have any questions, concerns, or would like a few words of encouragement, please don't hesitate to reach out (jcharrisonbooks@gmail.com).

Ending Each Session:

When you're finished with your yoga practice, take a few moments to meditate. This will help you to calm your mind and body and to integrate the benefits of your practice.

» Sit in a comfortable position in your chair. Close your eyes and take a few deep breaths. Focus on your breath, and let go of any thoughts or worries that come to mind.

» After a few minutes, you may want to try a simple meditation technique, such as focusing on a mantra or visualization. Or, you can simply sit quietly and enjoy the feeling of relaxation. For the meditation chapter, see page 239.

» When you're ready, open your eyes and slowly come back to the present moment. Take a few moments to appreciate the sense of relaxation and well-being that you've created.

Breathing Exercise: Three-Part Breath (3 min) p.37; **Warm-Up:** Side Neck Stretch (30s) p.45

Revolved Triangle	Wide Leg Forward	Half Moon Balance	Supported Sun Salutation	Supported Warrior II
30s (p. 184)	30s (p. 182)	30s (p. 192)	1 time (p. 188)	30s (p. 200)

Breathing Exercise: Lion's Breath (3 min) p.40; **Warm-Up:** Side Neck Stretch (30s) p.45

Reverse Warrior	Seated Locust	Upward Plank	Chair Dancer	Chair Downward Dog
30s (p. 172)	30s (p. 173)	30s (p. 178)	30s (p. 191)	30s (p. 176)

Breathing Exercise: Ocean Breath (3 min) p.38; **Warm-Up:** Shoulder Stretch (30s) p.45

Oblique Twists w/ Light Weight	Standing Back Arch	High-Leg Marches	Hovering Chair Pose	Chair Warrior III
30s (p. 220)	30s (p. 213)	30s (p. 216)	30s (p. 217)	30s (p. 183)

DAY 4: WEIGHT LOSS AND ENERGY

Breathing Exercise: Alternate Nostril (3 min) p.39; **Warm-Up:** Toe and Heel Lifts (30s) p.46

Mountain Climbers	Chair Push-Ups	Russian Twists	Chair Squat Jumps	Chair Plank
30s (p. 203)	30s (p. 209)	30s (p. 208)	30s (p. 210)	30s (p. 204)

DAY 5: FLEXIBILITY AND CORE STRENGTH

Breathing Exercise: Box Breathing (3 min) p.42; **Warm-Up:** Gentle Backbend (30s) p.46

Half Moon Balance	Chair Dancer	Chair Warrior I	Supported Warrior II	Seated Fish Pose
30s (p. 192)	30s (p. 191)	30s (p. 181)	30s (p. 200)	30s (p. 174)

DAY 6: LOWER BODY AND STABILITY

Breathing Exercise: Cooling Breath (3 min) p.41; **Warm-Up:** Gentle Twists (30s) p.44

Hovering Chair Pose	High Leg Marches	Russian Twists	Chair Plank	Chair Warrior III
30s (p. 217)	30s (p. 216)	30s (p. 208)	30s (p. 204)	30s (p. 183)

DAY 7: UPPER BODY AND POSTURE

Breathing Exercise: Diaphragmatic (3 min) p.36; **Warm-Up:** Side Neck Stretch(30s) p.45

Chair Downward Dog	Supported Warrior II	Chair Squat Jumps	Chair Push Ups	Revolved Head to Knee
30s (p. 176)	30s (p. 200)	30s (p. 210)	30s (p. 209)	30s (p. 171)

DAY 8: MOBILITY AND HEART HEALTH FOCUS

Breathing Exercise: Diaphragmatic (3 min) p.36; **Warm-Up:** Shoulder Stretch (40s) p.45

Revolved Triangle	High-Leg Marches	Half Moon Balance	Standing Back Arch	Chair Side Plank
40s (p. 184)	40s (p. 216)	40s (p. 192)	40s (p. 213)	40s (p. 218)

DAY 9: POSTURE AND BALANCE ENHANCEMENT

Breathing Exercise: Three-Part Breath (3 min) p.37; **Warm-Up:** Gentle Twists (40s) p.44

Reverse Warrior	Revolved Head to Knee	Standing Chair Eagle	Chair Dancer	Seated Locust
40s (p. 172)	40s (p. 171)	40s (p. 198)	40s (p. 191)	40s (p. 173)

DAY 10: FLEXIBILITY AND CORE STRENGTHENING

Breathing Exercise: Ocean Breath (3 min) p.38; **Warm-Up:** Seated Neck Rolls (40s) p.47

Seated Fish Pose	Half Moon Balance	Chair Warrior I	Standing Chair Eagle	Chair Downward Dog
40s (p. 174)	40s (p. 192)	40s (p. 181)	40s (p. 198)	40s (p. 176)

DAY 11: WEIGHT LOSS AND VITALITY

Breathing Exercise: Alternate Nostril (3 min) p.39; **Warm-Up:** Gentle Backbend (40s) p.46

Chair Warrior III	Seated Crescent Lunge	Mountain Climbers	Chair Squat Jumps	Chair Push-Ups
40s (p. 183)	40s (p. 186)	40s (p. 203)	40s (p. 210)	40s (p. 209)

DAY 12: STAMINA AND LOWER BODY FOCUS

Breathing Exercise: Box Breathing (3 min) p.42; **Warm-Up:** Toe and Heel Lifts (40s) p.46

Wide Leg Forward	Supported Sun Salutation	Chair Warrior I	Hovering Chair Pose	Chair Boat Pose
40s (p. 182)	1-2 times (p. 188)	40s (p. 181)	40s (p. 217)	40s (p. 206)

Breathing Exercise: Cooling Breath (3 min) p.41; **Warm-Up:** Gentle Backbend (40s) p.46

Revolved Triangle	Revolved Head to Knee	Half Moon Balance	Chair Warrior III	Chair Downward Dog
40s (p. 184)	40s (p. 171)	40s (p. 192)	40s (p. 183)	40s (p. 176)

Breathing Exercise: Lion's Breath (3 min) p.40; **Warm-Up:** Wrist & Ankle Rotation (40s) p.43

Supported Warrior II	Revolved Triangle	Russian Twists	Chair Side Plank	Supported Warrior Flow
40s (p. 200)	40s (p. 184)	40s (p. 208)	40s (p. 218)	1-2 times (p. 214)

Breathing Exercise: Diaphragmatic (3 min) p.36; **Warm-Up:** Seated Neck Rolls (45s) p.47

Oblique Twists w/Light Weight	Standing Back Arch	Chair Warrior III	Chair Boat Pose	Half Moon Balance
45s (p. 220)	45s (p. 213)	45s (p. 183)	45s (p. 206)	45s (p. 192)

Day 16: Posture and Balance

Breathing Exercise: Three-Part Breath (3 min) p.37; **Warm-Up:** Gentle Twists (45s) p.44

Reverse Warrior	Revolved Head to Knee	Standing Chair Eagle	Extended Side Angle	Chair Plank
45s (p. 172)	45s (p. 171)	45s (p. 198)	45s (p. 196)	45s (p. 204)

Day 17: Flexibility and Mobility

Breathing Exercise: Ocean Breath (3 min) p.38; **Warm-Up:** Wrist & Ankle Rotation (45s) p.43

Chair Squat Jumps	Chair Warrior I	Seated Fish Pose	Chair Downward Dog	Hovering Chair Pose
45s (p. 210)	45s (p. 181)	45s (p. 174)	45s (p. 176)	45s (p. 217)

Day 18: Weight Loss and Energy

Breathing Exercise: Alternate Nostril (3 min) p.39; **Warm-Up:** Gentle Twists (45s) p.44

Chair Boat Pose	Russian Twists	Mountain Climbers	Chair Squat Jumps	Chair Push-Ups
45s (p. 206)	45s (p. 208)	45s (p. 203)	45s (p. 210)	45s (p. 209)

Breathing Exercise: Box Breathing (3 min) p.42; **Warm-Up:** Shoulder Stretch (45s) p.45

Seated Humble Warrior	Extended Side Angle	Standing Chair Eagle	Seated Locust	Reverse Warrior
45s (p. 194)	45s (p. 196)	45s (p. 198)	45s (p. 173)	45s (p. 172)

DAY 20: BALANCE AND FLEXIBILITY

Breathing Exercise: Cooling Breath (3 min) p.41; **Warm-Up:** Side Neck Stretch (45s) p.45

Revolved Triangle	Chair Dancer	Wide Leg Forward	Chair Warrior III	Chair Downward Dog
45s (p. 184)	45s (p. 191)	45s (p. 182)	45s (p. 183)	45s (p. 176)

DAY 21: UPPER BODY AND POSTURE

Breathing Exercise: Lion's Breath (3 min) p.40; **Warm-Up:** Shoulder Stretch (45s) p.45

Chair Push Ups	Seated Fish Pose	Russian Twists	Chair Side Plank	Supported Warrior Flow
45s (p. 209)	45s (p. 174)	45s (p. 208)	45s (p. 218)	2-3 times (p. 214)

Day 22: Core Strengthening and Flexibility

Breathing Exercise: Diaphragmatic (3 min) p.36; **Warm-Up:** Gentle Backbend (50s) p.46

Standing Chair Eagle	Half Moon Balance	Chair Warrior I	Wide Leg Forward	Seated Fish Pose
50s (p. 198)	50s (p. 192)	50s (p. 181)	50s (p. 182)	50s (p. 174)

Day 23: Upper Body and Posture

Breathing Exercise: Three-Part Breath (3 min) p.37; **Warm-Up:** Toe and Heel Lifts (50s) p.46

Supported Sun Salutation	Seated Locust	Revolved Head to Knee	Chair Downward Dog	Reverse Warrior
2-3 times (p. 188)	50s (p. 173)	50s (p. 171)	50s (p. 176)	50s (p. 172)

Day 24: Balance and Heart Health

Breathing Exercise: Ocean Breath (3 min) p.38; **Warm-Up:** Seated Neck Rolls (50s) p.47

Standing Chair Eagle	Chair Dancer	Oblique Twists w/ Light Weight	High-Leg Marches	Hovering Chair Pose
50s (p. 198)	50s (p. 191)	50s (p. 220)	50s (p. 216)	50s (p. 217)

DAY 25: WEIGHT LOSS AND ENERGY

Breathing Exercise: Alternate Nostril (3 min) p.39; **Warm-Up:** Gentle Twists (50s) p.44

Mountain Climbers	Chair Push Ups	Upward Plank	Chair Squat Jumps	Russian Twists
50s (p. 203)	50s (p. 209)	50s (p. 178)	50s (p. 210)	50s (p. 208)

DAY 26: MOBILITY AND LOWER BODY FOCUS

Breathing Exercise: Box Breathing (3 min) p.42; **Warm-Up:** Wrist & Ankle Rotation (50s) p.43

Revolved Triangle	Extended Side Angle	Chair Boat Pose	Supported Warrior Flow	High Leg Marches
50s (p. 184)	50s (p. 196)	50s (p. 206)	2-3 times (p. 214)	50s (p. 216)

DAY 27: FLEXIBILITY AND BALANCE

Breathing Exercise: Cooling Breath (3 min) p.41; **Warm-Up:** Side Neck Stretch (50s) p.45

Half Moon Balance	Mountain Climbers	Chair Warrior III	Crescent Lunge	Chair Downward Dog
50s (p. 192)	50s (p. 203)	50s (p. 183)	50s (p. 186)	50s (p. 176)

Diaphragmatic Breathing	Warm-up	Review and practice	Closing
	Choose two of your favorite warm-ups to revisit	Choose your favorite poses to revisit	Relaxation and reflection session
3 minutes (p. 36)	50s each.	50s each.	

Week-by-Week Guide

Welcome to the 28-Day Advanced Flex Plan for Chair Yoga, here is how to get the most from this program over the next 28 days.

Getting Started:

» **Breathing and Warm-Up:** Before you begin, choose 1 breathing and 1 warm-up exercise, from Chapter Three (page 35), to start each day.

» **Choose Your Poses:** Each day, pick 4 or 5 poses that feel comfortable and enjoyable.

» **Flexibility in Your Routine:** Feel free to vary your poses daily. Adjust the duration to suit your energy levels and comfort.

» **Proceed at Your Pace:** Once your poses are selected, you're ready to continue with the program at a pace that feels right for you.

Remember: This journey is all about your wellness and flexibility, tailored to your unique needs and preferences. Let's take this step together, embracing health and joy at every turn!

28-DAY ADVANCED FLEX PLAN CHAIR YOGA PROGRAM

Week 1:

» Duration per Pose: 30 seconds.

» Daily Session Length: Start with 15 minutes.

» Focus: Introduce advanced stretches and strengthening exercises with increased range of motion.

» Breathing Exercises: Begin and end with diaphragmatic breathing.

Week 2:

» Duration per Pose: 40 seconds.

» Daily Session Length: Aim for Aim for 18-20 minutes.

» Focus: Greater emphasis on deep stretches and stronger balance poses.

» Breathing Exercises: Three-Part Breath for relaxation before and after the session.

Week 3:

» Duration per Pose: 45 seconds.

» Daily Session Length: Maintain at 20 minutes.

» Focus: Integrate complex standing poses using the chair for support, and incorporate active movements.

» Breathing Exercises: Ocean Breath (Ujjayi Pranayama) for focus.

Week 4:

» Duration per Pose: 50 seconds.

» Daily Session Length: Extend to 22-25 minutes.

» Focus: A comprehensive and challenging sequence, including all learned poses with advanced modifications.

» Breathing Exercises: Alternate nostril breathing to enhance relaxation.

> *The body benefits from movement, and the mind benefits from stillness.*
>
> – Sakyong Mipham

CHAPTER 7
MEDITATION AND CHAIR YOGA MADE EASY

Integrating meditation into your chair yoga routine offers a profound benefit, especially as we age. Meditation is a practice of focusing the mind on specific thoughts or experiences, a proven method for achieving a state of deep peace and relaxation. This mental discipline has roots stretching back thousands of years across various cultures, aimed at enhancing self-awareness, concentration, and spiritual growth. For seniors, the regular incorporation of meditation into daily life can be transformative, promoting mental clarity and a significant improvement in quality of life.

Research highlights meditation's ability to fortify neural pathways in the brain, crucial for memory retention and cognitive function, helping to mitigate age-related memory decline. Moreover, it boosts mood by increasing the production of serotonin and dopamine, the brain's natural feel-good chemicals. By consistently practicing meditation, you can also manage stress, lower levels of cortisol, the stress hormone, and maintain a serene and balanced mindset in everyday activities.

Meditation isn't just a practice, it's a transformation. As seniors, embracing meditation can be one of the most empowering decisions you make for your health and well-being. Keep this simple, remember this: meditation is about focusing the mind, and gently guiding your thoughts to create a haven of peace and clarity within you. This is not about becoming a Zen master overnight; it's about taking small, consistent steps towards a calmer, more centered you.

Unlocking a World of Benefits for Seniors

Stress Reduction: Stress isn't just a feeling; it's a physical response that can exacerbate health issues. Meditation is your secret weapon against this. It activates your body's relaxation response, helping reduce blood pressure and cortisol levels. Imagine feeling more at peace each day, with a heart that beats calmly and steadily.

Sharper Mind: Forgetfulness might seem like an inevitable part of aging, but meditation can help you sharpen your mind. It's like a workout for your brain, improving focus, attention, and memory. Picture your mind as a muscle that gets stronger and more resilient with each meditation session.

Emotional Resilience: Life's golden years should be just that – golden. Meditation helps in warding off feelings of loneliness or sadness, fostering a more positive and joyful outlook on life. It's about finding that inner strength and contentment, no matter what the day brings.

Pain Management: Many seniors struggle with chronic pain, but meditation can change your relationship with it. By focusing your mind, you can alter the way your body perceives pain, making it more manageable. It's about taking control, and not letting pain dictate your life.

<u>**Restful Sleep**</u>: Those nights of tossing and turning? Meditation can help. By calming your mind, you pave the way for deeper, more restful sleep. Imagine waking up each morning feeling refreshed and rejuvenated.

<u>**Improved Balance and Mobility**</u>: Meditation enhances body awareness, which in turn can improve balance and prevent falls. It's about being in tune with your body, moving through life with grace and confidence.

Incorporating meditation into your life is like planting a seed that grows into a tree of peace, resilience, and wellness. It's never too late to start. Each moment of mindfulness is a step towards a more vibrant, healthier you. Embrace this journey with an open heart and watch as your golden years become enriched with profound tranquility and joy.

Meditation: Your time, Your place

Choosing the right spot for meditation is key. Look for a quiet, peaceful area in your home where you can sit undisturbed. This could be a cozy corner or a spot with a pleasant view. The goal is to have a dedicated space that signals to your mind, "It's time to relax and focus." Consistency in your chosen spot helps in building a routine.

As for sitting, comfort is crucial. Use a sturdy chair that supports your back. Sit with your feet flat on the ground, hands resting gently in your lap. If needed, add cushions for extra support. The aim is to maintain a posture that's relaxed yet alert, ensuring you can focus without discomfort. Remember, in meditation, your comfort is the pathway to deeper focus and relaxation.

The perfect time to practice meditation is when it seamlessly fits into your routine, making it a sustainable and enjoyable habit. Here's the key: choose a time when you can be calm and undistracted, ensuring you get the most out of your practice.

Morning: Many find the early morning ideal, as the world is still quiet, allowing you to start your day with a clear, focused mind. It sets a positive tone for the day ahead.

Lunchtime or Breaks: A brief meditation session during lunch or on a break can be a great way to reset, especially if you're feeling stressed or overwhelmed.

Evening: If you need a way to unwind after a long day, evening meditation can be perfect. It helps you relax, let go of the day's stress, and improve sleep quality.

Before Bed: A short meditation before bed can aid in releasing the day's tensions, preparing your mind and body for a restful night's sleep.

Remember, the best time is when you can be consistent. Even just 5-10 minutes daily can make a significant impact. And don't forget, it's not just about fitting meditation into your schedule, but also embracing it as a moment of peace and self-care in your busy life. Let it be your personal retreat, a time when you prioritize your well-being and mental clarity.

To get you started with meditating I have included six different types of meditation practices that you can explore along with your chair yoga sessions.

Steps:

1. Choose a stable and comfortable place to sit (be it a chair, or bench). Ensure you're supported, not slouching or leaning. Place the soles of your feet flat on the ground.

2. Keep your back straight but relaxed, maintaining its natural curve. Let your head and shoulders rest naturally atop your spine.

3. Let your upper arms align with your body, then rest your hands on your legs. Find the middle ground—neither too far forward nor back.

4. Lower your chin slightly and allow your gaze to fall gently forward. You can close your eyes or keep them half-open, without focusing on anything specific.

5. Begin to Relax. Take a moment to relax into your position. Shift your attention to your breath or bodily sensations.

6. Notice the sensation of air moving in and out, choosing a point of focus (nose, belly, or chest). Mentally note "breathing in" and "breathing out."

7. When your mind wanders, gently bring your focus back to your breath. There's no need to stop thoughts, just return to your breathing.

8. If you need to move or scratch an itch, pause first. Choose intentionally when to adjust. Let thoughts and distractions come and go without engagement. Return to your breath each time without judgment.

9. When ready, gently lift your gaze (or open your eyes). Take in the sounds around you, feel your body, and acknowledge your thoughts and emotions. Pause, reflecting on how you wish to proceed with your day.

KEY TIP

Extend Mindfulness Beyond Meditation: Incorporate mindfulness into daily activities to deepen your awareness and presence in every moment.

BODY SCAN MEDITATION

Steps:

1. To get started lie down on your back on a comfortable surface. Ensure your body is in a straight line with arms resting at your sides, palms facing up. If lying down is uncomfortable, you can also do this seated in a chair.

2. Gently close your eyes to minimize distractions. This helps you focus more on internal sensations.

3. Breathe deeply and slowly a few times to initiate relaxation. Inhale through your nose, and exhale through your mouth, letting go of tension with each breath out.

4. **Start with Your Feet:** Focus your attention on your feet. Notice any sensations—warmth, coolness, pressure, tingling, or perhaps nothing at all. Breathe into your feet; as you exhale, imagine any tension melting away.

5. **Move to Your Legs:** Shift your focus up to your legs—calves, knees, and thighs. Observe any feelings or discomfort. With each exhale, release tension and let your legs relax completely.

6. **Notice Your Lower Back and Pelvis:** Bring awareness to your lower back and pelvis area. Breathe into these regions, relaxing muscles and releasing pressure as you exhale.

7. **Focus on Your Abdomen and Chest:** Pay attention to your abdomen and chest. Feel the rise and fall with each breath. Allow any tightness to dissolve with your out-breaths.

8. **Relax Your Shoulders and Neck:** Move your awareness to your shoulders and neck. These areas often hold a lot of stress. Breathe into them, and let the tension flow out as you breathe out.

9. **Pay Attention to Your Hands and Arms:** Notice any sensations in your hands and arms. Breathe in, directing your breath to these areas, and relax them fully as you breathe out.

BODY SCAN MEDITATION

Steps:

10. **Observe Your Face and Head:** Finally, focus on your face and head. Relax your jaw, cheeks, eyes, forehead, and the top of your head. Breathe in calmness and exhale any tension.

11. **Whole Body Awareness:** Expand your attention to include your whole body. Take a few deep breaths, feeling as if your entire body is breathing. With each exhale, release any remaining tension.

12. When you're ready, slowly bring movement back into your body by wiggling your fingers and toes. Gently open your eyes. Take a moment to notice how your body feels as a whole. Sit up slowly and transition back to your day.

KEY TIPS

Be Gentle with Yourself: If your mind wanders or if you lose focus, gently redirect your attention back to the body part you were focusing on.

Don't Rush: Move through each part of the body without hurry, allowing yourself to fully experience the sensations and relaxation.

WALKING MEDITATION

Steps:

1. Find a quiet, safe space where you can walk, either a path near your home or where you feel comfortable. This could be indoors or outdoors. The path doesn't need to be long, but it should allow you to walk without obstacles.

2. Stand at the start of your path. Close your eyes for a moment and set an intention for your practice. It could be anything that speaks to your current feelings, desires, or needs. It might be a word or a short phrase, such as "peace," "gratitude," "healing," or "being present." Your intention should resonate with you personally, reflecting something you wish to cultivate or acknowledge within yourself during the meditation. Take a few deep breaths to center yourself.

3. Gently open your eyes, maintaining a soft gaze. Be conscious of your surroundings but try to keep your focus inward.

4. Pay attention to your feet touching the ground. Feel the sensations in your soles as you lift one foot, move it forward, and place it down.

5. Begin to walk at a slower pace than usual. With each step, note the lifting, moving, and placing of each foot. This deliberate pace helps enhance awareness.

6. Sync your breathing with your steps, if possible. This might mean taking a step with each inhale and another with each exhale. Find a rhythm that feels natural to you.

7. Notice the sounds around you, the feel of the air on your skin, and anything you can see or smell. Acknowledge these sensations without getting attached to them.

8. If your mind wanders to other thoughts, gently bring your attention back to the act of walking and breathing. The goal is to stay present with each step and breath.

9. After completing your walk, stand still for a moment to reflect. Close your eyes and take a few deep breaths. Notice any sensations in your body or changes in your mind. Reflect on the sense of calm and presence you've cultivated.

10. **Open your eyes and gently transition back into your day, carrying the mindfulness and calmness with you.**

KEY TIPS

<u>Stay Relaxed</u>: Keep your body relaxed as you walk. Let your arms swing slightly if it feels natural.

<u>Use a Mantra</u>: If it helps, silently repeat a mantra or phrase with each step, such as "in" and "out" with your breaths, to help maintain focus.

<u>Adjust Your Pace</u>: The speed of your walking can vary based on what feels most conducive to mindfulness for you. Experiment with what helps you stay most present.

PRO TIP

"Keep a Meditation Journal"

After meditating, spend a few minutes reflecting on your experience and jotting down any insights, challenges, or feelings. A journal can track your progress and deepen your understanding of your meditation journey.

LOVING-KINDNESS MEDITATION

Steps:

1. Choose a quiet and comfortable place to sit. You can sit in a chair with your feet flat on the ground. Ensure your back is straight but relaxed.

2. Gently close your eyes. Take a few deep breaths to relax. With each exhale, release any tension you're holding.

3. Start by focusing on a feeling of warmth and kindness towards yourself. You might visualize a gentle, warm light enveloping you or recall a moment when you felt loved and cared for.

4. Silently repeat phrases of loving-kindness towards yourself. Common phrases include:

May I be happy.

May I be healthy.

May I be safe.

May I live with ease.

5. Bring to mind someone you love deeply. Imagine directing feelings of warmth and kindness towards them. Silently recite the same phrases of loving-kindness towards this person.

6. Gradually extend your circle of kindness to include:

   » A good friend

   » A neutral person (someone you neither like nor dislike)

   » A difficult person (no need to start with the most difficult person)

Steps:

7. Finally, extend loving-kindness to all beings everywhere, without limitation.

8. For each new recipient, visualize them clearly and recite your phrases of loving-kindness. Try to genuinely wish them well and feel the warmth of your kindness extending to them.

9. After you have extended loving-kindness to all beings, sit quietly for a moment. Notice the feelings in your heart and body. Often, practitioners feel a sense of warmth, openness, or connectedness.

10. When you're ready, gently open your eyes. Take a moment to transition back into your day, carrying the feelings of loving-kindness with you.

KEY TIPS

<u>Be Patient</u>: Cultivating loving-kindness can take time, especially if you're dealing with feelings of self-criticism or resentment towards others.

<u>Genuine Wishes</u>: Aim for sincerity in your wishes. It's not just about repeating the phrases but truly wishing well for yourself and others.

<u>Use Custom Phrases</u>: Feel free to adapt the phrases to better suit you or to address specific wishes for yourself and others.

VISUALIZATION MEDITATION

Steps:

1. Find a spot where you can sit or lie down comfortably without interruptions. Ensure your environment is conducive to relaxation and focus.

2. Sit in a comfortable position with your back straight but relaxed, or lie down if you prefer. Use cushions or blankets as needed to support your posture.

3. Gently close your eyes. Take deep, slow breaths to relax your body. With each exhale, consciously release tension from your muscles.

4. Think about what you wish to achieve with your visualization. It could be a state of mind, like peace or happiness, or a specific goal you're working toward.

5. Begin to picture a scene in your mind that embodies your intention. This could be a place where you feel completely at peace, like a beach at sunset, a serene forest, or a cozy, safe space.

6. Make the visualization as vivid as possible by involving all your senses. See the colors and shapes, hear the sounds, smell the scents, feel the textures, and taste any flavors. For example, if you're visualizing a beach, feel the warmth of the sun on your skin, hear the waves crashing, smell the saltwater, and taste the fresh air.

7. As you deepen into the visualization, try to genuinely feel the emotions associated with your scene. Embrace the calm, joy, or satisfaction your visualization brings.

8. Spend several minutes immersed in your visualization, allowing the scene to evolve naturally. If your mind wanders, gently bring your focus back to your visualization.

9. When you feel ready to end your meditation, slowly bring your awareness back to the present. Take a few deep breaths and start to move your fingers and toes.

10. Gently open your eyes. Take a moment to transition back into your surroundings. Reflect on the experience and any feelings or insights that arose.

11. Try to maintain the sense of calm, focus, or well-being you cultivated during your visualization as you go about your day.

KEY TIPS

Flexibility: Your visualization can change and evolve; there's no need to stick rigidly to the first image that comes to mind. Let your imagination flow freely.

Practice Regularly: Like any form of meditation, the benefits of visualization grow with regular practice. Make it a part of your daily routine for the best results.

Use Guided Visualizations: If you find it challenging to maintain a visualization on your own, consider using guided visualization recordings that can help lead you through the process.

MANTRA MEDITATION

Steps:

1. Choose a peaceful place where you won't be disturbed. Sitting in a dedicated meditation space can enhance your practice, but any quiet spot will do.

2. Sit in a comfortable position with your back straight. Ensure your posture is alert yet relaxed.

3. Select a mantra that resonates with you. It can be a traditional Sanskrit phrase like **"Om Mani Padme Hum"** (the jewel is in the lotus) or a simple word or phrase in any language that holds personal significance, such as **"peace,"** **"love,"** or **"I am calm."**

4. Gently close your eyes to minimize external distractions. This will help you focus inwardly and on the repetition of your mantra.

5. Take a few deep breaths to relax your body and mind. With each exhale, release any tension you're holding.

6. Silently repeat your mantra in your mind or whisper it softly. Your focus should be on the sound and vibration of the mantra as you recite it.

7. Continue to repeat your mantra at a pace that feels natural to you. There's no need to rush; allow the repetition to flow smoothly and steadily.

8. If you find your mind wandering to other thoughts, gently redirect your attention back to your mantra. The act of noticing distractions and returning to your mantra is part of the meditation process.

9. If you're concerned about time, set a timer for the duration you wish to meditate before you begin. This way, you can let go of the concern for time and fully immerse yourself in the practice.

10. When your meditation session is over, slowly cease the repetition of your mantra. Take a few deep breaths and gently bring your awareness back to your surroundings.

Steps:

11. Before opening your eyes, take a moment to notice the state of your mind and how you feel after the meditation. Acknowledge the peace and calm you've cultivated.

12. Open your eyes and take a moment to adjust. Move gently as you transition back to your daily activities, carrying the tranquility of your meditation with you.

KEY TIPS

<u>Consistency Is Key</u>: Regular practice enhances the benefits of Mantra Meditation. Aim to meditate at the same time each day to establish a routine.

<u>Be Patient</u>: It might take some time to notice the profound effects of your practice. Approach your meditation with patience and without expectation.

<u>Personalize Your Practice</u>: Feel free to adjust the length of your meditation sessions according to your comfort and schedule. Even a few minutes of dedicated practice can be beneficial.

Self-care is how you take your power back.

– Lalah Delia

CHAPTER 8
THE ESSENTIAL GUIDE TO
NUTRITION & CHAIR YOGA

Your Power Source in Senior Years

As we step into our senior years, it's time to turn a new page in our health story. Nutrition isn't just about eating; it's about fueling your life with the right energy. You might think it's too late to make changes, but I'm here to tell you it's not. Small shifts in your diet can lead to big wins in your health and vitality.

Nutrition's Impact: Why It's Crucial in Later Life

Remember, as we age, our bodies change. Our metabolism slows down, our digestive system may not be as efficient, and we might have different health concerns. But here's the good news: with the right nutrition, you can bolster your immune system, keep your bones strong, maintain your muscle mass, and feel more energetic. It's not just about adding years to your life, but life to your years!

THE BUILDING BLOCKS OF YOUR DIET

Let's talk about nutrition in a way that makes sense – no jargon, just straightforward facts. Your body is like a complex machine, and the food you eat is its fuel. Getting the right balance of nutrients is essential, but it doesn't have to be complicated. It's about getting back to basics and understanding the foundation of a healthy diet. These core principles are your allies in maintaining vitality and strength. Let's unravel these building blocks of nutrition, making each one simple and approachable. Whether it's the type of food you eat or the amount you consume, each element plays a crucial role in your overall health.

Let's simplify and look at what really matters:

Carbohydrates: Your Body's Primary Energy Source

Think of carbs as your body's main fuel. They break down into glucose (sugar in your blood), giving you the energy to keep moving.

Choose Wisely: Opt for whole grains like brown rice or whole wheat, and don't forget fiber-rich fruits and veggies. These carbs are processed more slowly, providing a steady energy supply without the sugar spikes.

Whole Grains	Fiber-rich fruits
Brown rice, quinoa, whole wheat bread.	Apples, berries (such as blueberries or strawberries), oranges.

Proteins: The Building Blocks of Muscle and More

Protein isn't just for bodybuilders. It's crucial for repairing tissues, making hormones, and maintaining muscle mass – especially important as you age.

Quality Counts: Lean meats, fish, beans, and nuts are excellent choices. They provide essential amino acids without excess fat. Quality proteins are essential for maintaining and not losing muscle as you age.

Lean meats	Beans and legumes	Nuts and seeds
Chicken breast, turkey, lean cuts of beef.	Black beans, lentils, chickpeas.	Almonds, walnuts, pumpkin seeds.

Fats: Don't Fear Them, Understand Them

Fats have a bad reputation, but good fats are vital for brain health, energy, and absorbing vitamins.

Go for the Good Fats: Focus on unsaturated fats found in avocados, olive oil, and fatty fish like salmon. These can help reduce the risk of heart disease.

Avocados	Olive oil	Fatty fish
A great source of healthy monounsaturated fats.	Ideal for dressing salads or light cooking.	Salmon, mackerel, and sardines are high in omega-3 fatty acids.

THE BUILDING BLOCKS OF YOUR DIET

Vitamins and Minerals: Your Secret Weapons

Think of them as your health's cheerleaders. Vitamin C boosts your immune system, Vitamin D is essential for bones, and B vitamins are key for energy.

Vitamins: From Vitamin A to Zinc, these little guys help keep your body functioning at its best. Focus on getting a colorful variety of fruits and vegetables to cover your bases.

Minerals: They're like the nuts and bolts keeping your body in top shape. Calcium and magnesium strengthen bones, iron is vital for healthy blood, and potassium helps control blood pressure.

Vitamin-rich fruits	Mineral-rich vegetables
Kiwi (rich in Vitamin C), bananas (potassium), cantaloupe (Vitamin A).	Spinach (iron and magnesium), broccoli (calcium and Vitamin K), sweet potatoes (Vitamin A and potassium).

Portion Control: Balance is Key

Eating the right amounts is just as important as eating the right foods. Listen to your body's hunger cues and remember, moderation is your friend.

A balanced plate: Half filled with vegetables, one-quarter with lean protein, and one-quarter with whole grains.

Snack portions: A small handful of nuts, a piece of fruit, or a cup of yogurt.

Fiber: more than just a dietary component

Fiber is a crucial player in your digestive health. Acting like a natural cleanser, fiber helps keep your digestive system running smoothly and efficiently. Often overlooked, fiber keeps your digestive system happy and can help manage blood sugar levels.

Incorporate fiber into your diet with choices like:

Whole grains, oats, fruits (like apples and pears), vegetables (like carrots and green beans), beans and legumes, such as lentils and chickpeas, are also excellent sources of fiber.

Hydration: The Elixir of Life

Water is crucial. It keeps everything running smoothly in your body. Not a fan of plain water? Try adding a slice of lemon or cucumber for a refreshing twist.

Water: The most straightforward and effective hydrator.

Herbal teas: Such as chamomile or peppermint, which are hydrating and can have additional health benefits.

Infused water: Adding cucumber, lemon, or berries to water for flavor.

Why Strengthening Bones and Muscles is Crucial

As we navigate our senior years, focusing on bone and muscle health isn't just a health recommendation; it's a necessity for active, independent living. Strong bones reduce the risk of fractures, and well-maintained muscles are essential for mobility, balance, and even simple daily tasks.

Bones: The Framework of Your Body: With age, bones can become more fragile due to a natural decline in bone density. A diet rich in calcium and vitamin D plays a critical role in maintaining bone strength and preventing osteoporosis.

Muscles: Your Source of Strength and Mobility: Muscle mass naturally decreases with age. However, consuming adequate protein and engaging in regular physical activity, like chair yoga, can help preserve and even build muscle strength.

Nutritional Keys for Bone and Muscle Health

Calcium	Vitamin D	Protein
It's the cornerstone for strong bones. Dairy products like milk and cheese, leafy greens like kale, and fortified foods are excellent sources.	Essential for calcium absorption, vitamin D can be obtained from the sun, but food sources like fatty fish, egg yolks, and fortified foods play a vital role, especially in colder climates or for those with limited sun exposure.	Crucial for muscle repair and growth. Options like lean meats, fish, beans, and nuts not only provide protein but are also packed with other nutrients beneficial for overall health.

Making It Pratical

Incorporating these nutrients into your daily meals can be both simple and delicious. Start your day with a Greek yogurt parfait, enjoy a spinach salad for lunch, and have grilled salmon for dinner. Snacks like a handful of almonds or cottage cheese can also be a tasty way to get your daily dose of bone and muscle-supporting nutrients.

Remember, what you eat directly impacts the strength and resilience of your bones and muscles. By choosing the right foods, you're not just eating; you're investing in your ability to live actively and independently.

Discover the Key to Longevity: Heart & Gut Health for Seniors

Maintaining a healthy heart and digestive system is more than just managing health; it's about enhancing the quality of life as you age. A strong heart ensures that your body gets the necessary nutrients and oxygen, while a well-functioning digestive system is key to absorbing these nutrients effectively. Together, they form the core of your well-being, influencing everything from energy levels to mood.

<u>Heart Health:</u> As we age, our heart requires more attention. Eating heart-healthy foods can help manage blood pressure, reduce cholesterol levels, and lower the risk of heart disease.

<u>Digestive System:</u> A robust digestive system aids in efficiently processing the food you eat, ensuring you reap the benefits of a nutritious diet. This is crucial for avoiding common age-related digestive issues.

Nutritional Strategies for a Happy Heart and Gut

Oats and Whole Grains

Rich in soluble fiber, they help lower cholesterol levels and provide a steady source of energy.

Probiotic Foods

Yogurt, kefir, and fermented foods like sauerkraut help maintain a healthy gut flora, crucial for good digestion.

Berries and Antioxidant-Rich Foods

These help reduce inflammation and support heart health. Blueberries, strawberries, and raspberries are not only delicious but also packed with heart-healthy nutrients.

Leafy Greens and Fibrous Vegetables

Foods like spinach, kale, and broccoli are great for the heart and the digestive system, offering essential nutrients and fiber.

Why Energy and Immunity are Crucial in Senior Years

In our senior years, having consistent energy and a strong immune system isn't just a luxury; it's essential for enjoying life to its fullest. Sustained energy helps us stay active, engaged, and independent, while a robust immune system is our first line of defense against illnesses. The good news? Your diet plays a pivotal role in bolstering both.

Sustained Energy: As metabolism naturally slows with age, choosing the right foods can help maintain steady energy levels throughout the day.

Robust Immunity: With age, the immune system can weaken. A nutrient-rich diet supports its functioning, helping you stay healthier and recover faster from illnesses.

Diet Tips for Sustained Energy and Immunity

Complex Carbohydrates for Long-Lasting Energy: Foods like sweet potatoes, brown rice, and whole grain bread provide a gradual release of energy, preventing spikes and crashes.

Lean Proteins for Strength and Stamina: Incorporate chicken, turkey, fish, and plant-based proteins like beans and lentils. These help repair and build tissues, contributing to overall vitality.

<u>Antioxidant-Rich Fruits and Vegetables for Immune Support:</u> Citrus fruits, berries, bell peppers, and leafy greens are loaded with vitamins C and E, which bolster the immune system.

 <u>Healthy Fats for Energy and Cell Health:</u> Avocados, nuts, and olive oil provide essential fatty acids, supporting cell health and energy production.

Practical Ways to Boost Energy and Immunity

Regular, Balanced Meals

Eating at consistent times helps regulate your energy levels. Include a mix of carbohydrates, proteins, and fats in each meal.

Stay Hydrated

Adequate hydration is key for energy and immune function. Aim for water, herbal teas, and hydrating foods like cucumbers and watermelon.

Snack Smart

Choose snacks that combine protein and fiber, like apple slices with almond butter or yogurt with berries, for an energy and immune-boosting lift.

By focusing on these dietary strategies, you're equipping your body with the tools it needs to maintain high energy levels and a resilient immune system. This isn't just about food; it's about fueling your body for a joyful, active life in your senior years.

CONCLUSION

"Age is no barrier. It's a limitation you put on your mind."

– Jackie Joyner-Kersee

As we wrap up our chair yoga journey, it's time to reflect briefly on what we've accomplished together. This book isn't just information; it's your roadmap to a life filled with energy and positivity, no matter your age.

You now understand how to practice chair yoga comfortably and safely, equipped with techniques that can transform your daily experiences. Imagine navigating your day with ease, finding joy in routine tasks, and being an inspiration in every gathering. Chair yoga is more than exercise; it's a path to independence, health, and an optimistic view of life.

Crafted with love and intention, this book aimed to light a spark within you—to show that chair yoga is a golden key accessible to all, customizable to your unique rhythm, and immensely rewarding. With every pose you master, you'll feel yourself growing stronger, your body becoming more supple, and your balance steadier. Each small victory on the mat mirrors a giant leap toward a life that's richer and more vibrant.

Chair yoga is not just a routine; it's a testament to your strength and ability to adapt. Begin with enthusiasm, leverage the tools you've learned, and believe in gradual progress. This journey is about patience, celebrating each achievement, and staying committed. Keep refining your practice as you advance, making it a cornerstone of your health.

Let this book be more than a guide; let it be the dawn of a commitment to a practice that enriches every corner of your existence. Step into the embrace of chair yoga with an open heart and let it infuse your life with its transformative energy. Here's to you—stepping boldly into a future filled with health, happiness, and the joy of living life to the fullest, one breath, one pose at a time.

Now that you've embarked on this incredible journey with me, discovering the ease and joy of chair yoga, you're equipped with all the tools you need to embrace a life full of movement, flexibility, and peace. It's your turn to pass the torch and illuminate the path for others seeking the same serenity and vitality you've found.

By sharing your genuine thoughts about "10 Min Chair Yoga for Seniors Over 60" on Amazon, you're not just leaving a review; you're guiding other seniors towards a gateway of transformation. Your words have the power to light the way for someone else in search of a brighter, more active, and joyful chapter in their life.

We're all part of a beautiful cycle of learning and teaching, giving and receiving. Your contribution by leaving a review keeps this cycle in motion, ensuring that the wisdom and benefits of chair yoga continue to enrich lives far and wide.

Thank you deeply for your support. The legacy of chair yoga thrives and expands with each story shared and each life touched – and you're playing a pivotal role in this beautiful journey.

Go to https://geni.us/ChairYogaBook or scan to leave your review on Amazon.

Your insights and experiences are invaluable, not just to us, but to the countless others on the cusp of discovering their own path to wellness through chair yoga. Together, we're not just practicing yoga; we're fostering a community of health, happiness, and shared knowledge. Thank you for being an essential part of this community and for helping to keep the spirit of chair yoga alive and flourishing!

REFERENCES

Bao, W., Sun, Y., Zhang, T., Zou, L., Wu, X., Wang, D., & Chen, Z. (2020). Exercise Programs for Muscle Mass, Muscle Strength and Physical Performance in Older Adults with Sarcopenia: A Systematic Review and Meta-Analysis. Aging and Disease, 11, 863 - 873. https://doi.org/10.14336/ad.2019.1012.

Bonura, K., & Tenenbaum, G. (2014). Effects of yoga on psychological health in older adults. Journal of physical activity & health, 11 7, 1334-41. https://doi.org/10.1123/jpah.2012-0365.

Fishman, L. (2021). Yoga and Bone Health. Orthopaedic Nursing, 40, 169 - 179. https://doi.org/10.1097/NOR.0000000000000757.

Ghahramani, A. (2014). The effect of the relaxation training on the general health and selected physical fitness factors affecting seniors balance. Asian journal of multidisciplinary studies, 3.

Law, S., Leung, A., & Xu, C. (2021). Is Yoga possible for elderly care? Geriatric Care. https://doi.org/10.4081/GC.2021.9815.

Marciniak, R., Sheardová, K., Čermaková, P., Hudeček, D., Šumec, R., & Hort, J. (2014). Effect of Meditation on Cognitive Functions in Context of Aging and Neurodegenerative Diseases. Frontiers in Behavioral Neuroscience, 8. https://doi.org/10.3389/fnbeh.2014.00017.

McArthur, C., Laprade, J., & Giangregorio, L. (2016). Suggestions for Adapting Yoga to the Needs of Older Adults with Osteoporosis.. Journal of alternative and complementary medicine, 22 3, 223-6. https://doi.org/10.1089/acm.2014.0397. McCaffrey, R., Park, J., Newman, D., & Hagen, D. (2014). The effect of chair yoga in older adults with moderate and severe Alzheimer's disease. Research in gerontological nursing, 7 4, 171-7. https://doi.org/10.3928/19404921-20140218-01.

Park, J., & McCaffrey, R. (2012). Chair yoga: benefits for community-dwelling older adults with osteoarthritis. Journal of gerontological nursing, 38 5, 12-22; quiz 24-5. https://doi.org/10.3928/00989134-20120410-01.

Park, J., Newman, D., McCaffrey, R., Garrido, J., Riccio, M., & Liehr, P. (2016). The Effect of Chair Yoga on Biopsychosocial Changes in English- and Spanish-Speaking Community-Dwelling Older Adults with Lower-Extremity Osteoarthritis. Journal of Gerontological Social Work, 59, 604 - 626. https://doi.org/10.1080/016 34372.2016.1239234.

Park, J., Tolea, M., Rosenfeld, A., Arcay, V., Karson, J., Lopes, Y., Small, K., & Galvin, J. (2018). FEASIBILITY AND EFFECTS OF CHAIR YOGA TO MANAGE DEMENTIA SYMPTOMS IN OLDER ADULTS. Innovation in Aging. https://doi.org/10.1093/GERONI/IGY023.1142.

REFERENCES

Yao, C., & Tseng, C. (2019). Effectiveness of Chair Yoga for Improving the Functional Fitness and Well-being of Female Community-Dwelling Older Adults With Low Physical Activities. Topics in Geriatric Rehabilitation, 35, 248 - 254. https://doi.org/10.1097/TGR.0000000000000242.

You, S., Hong, S., & Moon, K. (2013). Effects of Hatha Yoga Practice on the Elderly Having Chronic Back Pain Because of Computer Usage. The Journal of the Korea institute of electronic communication sciences, 8, 1121-1128. https://doi.org/10.13067/JKIECS.2013.8.7.1121.

Made in the USA
Columbia, SC
08 September 2024

42010198R00148